Some Blood and Heart related Diseases

Some Blood and Heart related Diseases

◆

Including some known risk factors
for the diseases.
Modifying the controllable risk factors.
Deep Vein Thrombosis (DVT) and Sickle
cell anemia.

Gabriel Ademola

iUniverse, Inc.
New York Bloomington Shanghai

Some Blood and Heart related Diseases
Including some known risk factors
for the diseases.
Modifying the controllable risk factors.
Deep Vein Thrombosis (DVT) and Sickle cell anemia.

iUniverse books may be ordered through booksellers or by contacting:

iUniverse
1663 Liberty Drive
Bloomington, IN 47403
www.iuniverse.com
1-800-Authors (1-800-288-4677)

Because of the dynamic nature of the Internet, any Web addresses or links contained in this book may have changed since publication and may no longer be valid.

The information, ideas, and suggestions in this book are not intended as a substitute for professional medical advice. Before following any suggestions contained in this book, you should consult your personal physician. Neither the author nor the publisher shall be liable or responsible for any loss or damage allegedly arising as a consequence of your use or application of any information or suggestions in this book.

ISBN: 978-0-595-51407-6 (pbk)
ISBN: 978-0-595-61886-6 (ebk)

Printed in the United States of America

For my wife and beautiful daughters

Contents

Part Two: The Heart

Part Three: Cardiovascular and Coronary Artery Diseases

Part Four: Some Diagnostic Tests and Checks

Part Five: Keeping your heart healthy

Part Six: Stress

Preface

This book was inspired from personal experience and that of some loved ones and friends. I have been around loved ones and friends that have had to live with and through the morbidity of interference with quality of live and creation of serious handicaps caused by cardiovascular and coronary artery diseases.

Almost all of these events are avoidable with appropriate lifestyle and choices modification, and by early diagnosis and specific treatment for individual cases.

The data for the book was compiled from variety of sources including discussions and interviews with administering physicians and data from free and public domain of on-line resources. However, this data is not intended to substitute or replace the professional advice of your physician. It is advisable to consult your doctor with any questions or concerns you may have regarding your health or condition.

Introduction

Cardiovascular Disease (CVD) encompasses all the diseases of the heart and surrounding blood vessels. Coronary artery Disease (CAD) is caused by accumulation of plaque and fatty deposits inside the arteries, resulting in decrease or blockage of blood flow to the heart muscles. Heart disease refers to a variety of medical conditions affecting the heart including heart attack, heart failure, and angina. Stroke is caused by either a blockage or rupture of the blood vessels leading to and from the brain. This prevents vital oxygen and nutrients from reaching the brain thereby starving cells and causing potentially irreparable damage.

These diseases are reported to be in the top league of known killer diseases worldwide. It is said that some controllable risk factors such as physical inactivity, overweight or obesity, high blood cholesterol, high blood pressure, diabetes, and smoking are all major influences in the development, progression, and severity of these diseases.

Prevention is still agreed to be the best weapon in the fight against these diseases.

Part One:

The Blood, Blood vessels, and some related diseases

What is blood?

Blood is the fluid circulating through the blood vessels in the body. It can also be termed the fluid of life. It contains Red blood cells (erythrocytes), White blood cells (leukocytes), Platelets (thrombocytes) and pale yellowish liquid called plasma. The most important component of the blood is believed to be the red blood cell, which contains haemoglobin; the oxygen-affinity protein that carries oxygen from the lungs to all parts of the body. The primary function of the white blood cells is to fight infection and there are several types of white blood cells, each with its own role in fighting bacterial, viral, fungal, and parasitic infections. The primary function of the platelets is blood clotting. They are much smaller in size than the other blood cells and they aggregate to form jelly clumps, plugging any hole in a blood vessel to stop bleeding.

Blood cells are said to be made in the bone marrow in a production and development process called hematopoiesis. The bone marrow is the soft, spongy material in the centre of the bones. Blood cells formed in the bone marrow start life as a stem cell. A stem cell (hematopoietic cell) is the initial phase of all blood cells. As the stem cells mature, several distinct cells such as red blood cells, white blood cells, and platelets evolve. Immature blood cells are called blasts. Some blasts are believed to stay in the marrow to mature while others travel to other parts of the body to develop into mature, functioning blood cells. Other organs and systems in the body also help regulate blood cells. The lymph nodes, spleen, and liver are said to help regulate the production, destruction, and differentiation of blood cells.

The blood flows through a system of arteries, capillaries and veins. Arteries carry blood away from the heart into the body and veins carry blood back to the heart. The vein walls are thinner and less elastic than the artery walls, and they contain one-way check valves to prevent the reverse flow of blood. The smallest blood vessels are the capillaries, which form a network in the body tissues and enable exchange of oxygen and nutrients within the individual cells in tissue.

The body produces enough blood to carryout life's function and when there is a shortfall it is called anaemia. Anaemia is not a disease but it is an ailment caused by some diseases and its cause should be investigated and treated. Most anaemia is from excessive blood loss such as in heavy menstrual periods, bleeding ulcers or bleeding cancer in the bowel. Diseases that reduce the production of red blood cells such as leukaemia and sickle cell disorder may also cause anaemia. Doctors may order a red blood count for symptoms of fatigue, dizziness or headache for diagnosis of anaemia; however, mild anaemia may not produce these symptoms. Thorough examination and x-ray maybe required to confirm the source of blood loss. A complete blood cell count (CBC) is a measurement of size, number, and maturity of the different blood cells in a specific volume of blood.

Blood Platelets

Platelets (thrombocytes) are tiny cells that circulate in the blood and whose function is to take part in the clotting process. Inside each platelet are granules, containing compounds that enhance the ability of the platelets to stick to each other and also to the surface of a damaged blood vessel wall.

Platelets are essential in the formation of blood clots to prevent haemorrhage (bleeding) from a ruptured blood vessel. Adequate numbers of normal functioning platelets are also needed to prevent leakage of red blood cells through blood vessel walls.

After injury that results in bleeding, muscles in the blood vessel wall contracts, reducing blood leakage. Platelets then stick together (aggregation) and hold unto the vessel wall. The coagulation factor is then activated, leading to the liquid blood becoming an insoluble gel or clot.

Reduced blood platelets count (thrombocytopenia)

This is when platelets are lost from circulation faster than they can be replaced from the bone marrows, where they are made. It can result from:

- A failure of platelets production or
- An increased rate of platelets removal from the blood.

The average life span of a platelet in the blood is about ten days and the platelets count in the circulating blood is normally between 150—400 million per millilitre of blood.

Effects of thrombocytopenia

The main effect of a reduced platelets count is an increased bleeding risk, but this rarely occurs until there are less than about 80—100 million per millilitre of blood. There is said to be a particular high risk of spontaneous bleeding once the count drops below 10 million per millilitre. Bleeding from the nose and gums is also common. More serious haemorrhage can also occur at the back of the eye (retina), sometimes threatening vision. The most serious and potentially fatal complication is spontaneous bleeding inside the head (intracranial) or from the gut lining (gastro-intestinal).

Causes of thrombocytopenia

Some false low platelets count can result from a blood sample test—some platelets may stick together in the presence of antibodies in the blood. These antibodies can also bind to a chemical that is tested in the laboratory, giving a false low platelets count. False low platelets count can also result if the blood sample is difficult to take and the blood then clots, using up some of the platelets. For this reason, caution is advised and it is helpful to repeat the test in different apparatus with different chemicals.

Real low platelets count can result from defective platelets production due to:

- Bone marrow failure (a problem in the bone marrow due to abnormal cells or abnormality in the cells that makeup the structural parts of the bone marrow).
- Metabolic disorder such as from kidney failure; alcohol abuse; and shortage of vitamin b12 or folic acid.
- Viral infection.
- Drugs side effects such as chemotherapy agents.
- Acute leukaemia or abnormal cancer cells, leading to bone marrow infiltration.
- Congenital or inherited abnormalities.

Real low platelets count can also be due to diminished platelet survival rate or loss of platelets from circulation due to the followings:

- Production of antibodies in response to some drugs such as in malaria or glandular fever treatment.
- Blood clotting disorders.
- Some blood disorders.
- Blood transfusion, causing platelets dilution.

- Enlarged spleen causing abnormal blood dilution factors (platelets build up outside the normal blood pool as in someone with very large spleen)

- Unknown cause (abnormal antibodies build up in a normal person resulting in low platelets count).

Investigation of this condition as with other blood disorder cases usually starts with the history of the symptoms or other medical problems. The physician would require that a blood sample be taken for tests and analysis. Other medical procedures might follow. The choice of treatment will depend on the severity of the low count; its apparent cause and any presence of bleeding. The management of acute bleeding also involves treatment of the underlying cause of the low platelets.

Please discuss fully with your doctor.

Increased Red blood cell count (polycythaemia)

This is when there are too many red blood cells in the blood. It is also called erythrocytosis.

Red blood cells are the major component of the blood and their main content is the oxygen-bearing protein called haemoglobin. Red blood cells have special doughnut-like shape, which allows them to bend and squeeze through the smallest of blood vessels. The number of red blood cells in the blood varies according to age and sex—with men reportedly having higher levels; and newborn babies having more than adults.

The main problem caused by polycythaemia is that the high number of red blood cells increases the blood's viscosity, thereby slowing or reducing blood flow to the tissues. And rarely, blood clots may form. The risk of clotting (thrombosis) increases with other risk factors for blood vessel disease such as:—high blood pressure, diabetes, high LDL blood cholesterol or previous clot history.

Absolute erythrocytosis (raised red cell mass and normal plasma volume) is when there is actual increase in red blood cells.

Apparent erythrocytosis (normal red cell mass and reduced plasma volume) is when there is no increase in red cells, but they are more concentrated.

Causes

Absolute primary erythrocytosis can be caused by abnormality within the red blood cells. This can be either:

- Congenital (present at birth)—red cell disorders causing enhanced erythropoietin production. (Erythropoietin is the hormone that regulates the red blood cell production) or

- Acquired (develops sometime after birth)—Abnormality of the red blood cells in the bone marrow.

Absolute secondary erythrocytosis can be caused by abnormality outside of the red blood cells. This can be:

- Congenital (present at birth)—inherited high erythropoietin levels; abnormal haemoglobin with increased oxygen affinity and decreased level of metabolite. Both conditions lead to less oxygen delivery to the body tissues and the body then responds by increasing the total quantity of haemoglobin and thus red blood cells.

- Acquired (develops sometime after birth)—conditions causing low oxygen levels such as chronic lung disease; some types of congenital heart disease and sleep apnoea; kidney disease; liver disease; tumours; abnormal blood vessels in the brain; endocrine (hormonal) disorders; and unknown cause (idiopathic erythrocytosis).

Apparent erythrocytosis can be caused by factors such as:

- Obesity (overweight)
- Use of diuretics (water removal pills)
- Fluid loss.
- Smoking.
- High blood pressure.
- High alcohol intake.
- Kidney disease.
- Stress.

The increase in cells may be temporary and resolve itself once the cause is addressed. However, any increase of cells should be monitored as it may indicate the start of a true erythrocytosis.

A raised red blood cell count most often develops from another disease and this is because a problem outside of the bone marrow stimulates the production of red blood cells. These can either be those that causes low oxygen levels in the blood, say, from a kidney artery blockage or lung disease; or those that causes enhanced erythropoietin production, say, from a tumour. If the cause of a raised red blood cell count is unknown, then continual monitoring will be required as this might have a medically significant cause manifesting later and requiring treatment.

Symptoms of polycythaemia

Some symptoms that can be a feature of increased red blood cell count may include:

- Headache.
- Blurred vision or patchy loss of vision.
- Confusion.
- A ruddy complexion.
- In extreme cases, stroke or even coma.

It is obvious that these symptoms are not exclusively for increased blood thickness and are often rather vague. Therefore, a battery of different tests will be used to decide if and why someone has erythrocytosis. An increase in red blood cell count might first show in a blood test result as:—an increase in red cell numbers; a rise in haemoglobin; or a rise in the packed cell volume (measurement of the volume of red cells in the blood).

For a confirmed abnormal result the doctor might review the patient's medical history, symptoms and other medications. Other diagnostic tests may also be performed.

Generally, treatment of polycythaemia is directed at the underlying cause and if a cure is apparently impossible, the doctor might decide on whether specific treatment to reduce the red cell count is required.

Leukemia (blood cancer)

This is a disease where the bone marrow produces large numbers of abnormal cells, resulting in the presence of unusually high numbers of abnormal white blood cells in the blood stream. Leukemia, which means "white blood" in Greek, is a form of cancer that begins in the blood-forming cells of the bone marrow. The abnormal white blood cells (leukocytes) in the blood can be so plentiful in some patients that the blood is said to actually have a whitish tinge.

Normally, the blood-forming (haematopoietic) cells of the bone marrow make leukocytes to defend the body against infectious organisms, such as viruses and bacteria. If some leukocytes are damaged and remain in an immature form, they become poor infection fighters that multiply excessively and do not die off as they should.

These damaged leukemic cells accumulate and lessen the production of oxygen-carrying red blood cells (erythrocytes), blood-clotting cells (platelets), and normal leukocytes. The surplus leukemic cells can overwhelm the bone marrow, enter the blood stream, and eventually invade the other parts of the body such as the lymph nodes; spleen; liver; and central nervous system (brain, spinal cord).

TYPES

Leukemia is classified according to the cell type affected and clinical course. The course may be acute (fast-growing and can overrun the body within a few weeks or months) or chronic (slow-growing and progressively worsens over the years). Leukemia is also classified according to the type of white blood cell that is multiplying. If the abnormal white blood cells are granulocytes (bacteria-destroying cells) or monocytes (macrophage-forming cells), the leukemia is categorized as myelogenous leukemia. But, if the abnormal blood cells arise from bone marrow lymphocytes (immune system cells), the cancer is called lymphocytic leukemia.

There are many different types of leukemia but the following four types are reportedly most common:

- Acute lymphocytic leukemia (ALL).

- Acute myelogenous leukemia (AML).

- Chronic lymphocytic leukemia (CLL).

- Chronic myelogenous leukemia (CML).

Acute lymphocytic leukemia (ALL)—also known as acute lymphoblastic leukemia—is a malignant disease caused by the abnormal growth and development of early nongrannular white blood cells, or lymphocytes. The leukemia is said to originate in the blast cells of the bone marrow (B-cells), thymus (T-cells), and lymph nodes. It occurs predominantly in children, and is said to peak at four years of age.

Acute myelogenous leukemia (AML)—also known as acute nonlymphocytic leukemia—is the most common form of adult leukemia, with reported average age at diagnosis of about sixty-five years. More men are said to be affected than women. Fortunately, because of recent advances in treatment, AML reportedly can be kept in remission (lessening degree of the disease) in high proportion of adults who undergo appropriate therapy.

Chronic lymphocytic leukemia (CLL)—is a disease of older adults and is said to be very rare amongst people who are younger than fifty years of age. More men are reportedly affected than women. CLL is thought to result from the gradual accumulation of mature, long-lived lymphocytes. Therefore, it is caused by extreme longevity and build-up of malignant cells and not so much as by overgrowth. The rate of accumulation varies in patients, but the extensive tumour burden is said to eventually cause complications in all cases of CLL. The disease usually is detected accidentally during a doctor's examination for an unrelated complaint.

Chronic myelogenous leukemia (CML)—is also known as myeloproliferative disorder—and is a disease in which bone marrow cells proliferate (multiply) outside of the bone marrow tissue. CML is reported to occur in adults, with the median age of about sixty-seven years. It occasionally affects people in their 20s, but it is rare in the very young. The early disease is said to be without symptoms and is discovered accidentally. CML is also said to be easily diagnosed, since it has a genetic peculiarity, or marker, that is readily identifiable under a microscope.

SYMPTOMS

Early signs of leukemia is said to be often vague or non-specific. Although signs and symptoms vary for each type of leukemia and for individuals, there are some general features and some symptoms of leukemia may include:

- Fatigue or general feeling of bodily discomfort.

- Weakness.

- Abnormal bleeding or excessive bruising.

- Weight loss.

- Reduced exercise tolerance.

- Infection and fever.

- Bone or joint pain.

- Abdominal pain or bloating; caused by enlarged spleen (splenomegaly) and enlarged liver (hepatomegaly). Such fullness may be felt by the physician during physical examination.

- Enlarged spleen and/or enlarged liver.

The mentioned symptoms are not exclusively for leukemia; therefore it is advisable to consult with your doctor for diagnosis and treatment.

Chronic leukemia is said to often go undetected for many years until it is identified in a routine blood test. Most symptoms of acute leukemia are also said to be caused by lack of normal blood cells, which is due to overcrowding of the blood-forming bone marrow by leukemia cells.

After testing the patient's blood; signs of specific blood abnormalities may be noted, such as:

- Anemia—a low number of red blood cells within the blood.

- Leukopenia—low numbers of normal white blood cells in the blood that may increase risk of infection.

- Neutropenia—too few mature neutrophils; the mature bacteria-destroying white blood cells that contain small particles, or granules.

- Thrombocytopenia—a low number of blood-clotting platelets that can result in excessive bruising, abnormal bleeding, or frequent bleeding of the nose or gums.

- Thrombocytosis—a high number of platelets. Some patients may exhibit thrombocytosis and their platelets may not clot properly, causing bruising and bleeding difficulties.

Leukemia that has spread to the brain may produce central nervous system effects such as headaches, seizures, weakness, blurred vision, balance difficulties, or vomiting.

Certain forms of leukemia is said to produce more distinct symptoms such as:

- Swollen, painful or bleeding gums.

- Pigmented (coloured) rash-like spots

- Chloromas (granulocytic sarcomas—collections of tumorous cells within the skin or other body parts; if it has spread to the skin or other organs).

- Shortness of breath

- Coughing or feeling of suffocation.

- Swelling of the head and arms—SVC syndrome. If an overgrown thymus presses upon the superior vena cava (SVC), the large vein that carries blood from the head and arms back to the heart, this may produce SVC syndrome.

CAUSES

Many cellular changes associated with leukemia is said to have been researched but it is still unknown why these changes occur. However certain risk factors are believed to be involved. It is now known that all cancers—including leukemia, begin as a mutation in the genetic material—the DNA (deoxyribonucleic acid)—within body cells. Leukemia is thought to begin when one or more white blood cells experience DNA loss or damage. Those errors are copied and passed on to subsequent generations of cells. The abnormal leukemic cells are said to remain in an immature blast cell form that never matures properly. They do not die off like normal cells, but tend to multiply and accumulate within the body.

DNA errors may also occur in the form of translocations—damage produced when part of one chromosome becomes displaced and attached to another chromosome. Translocation is said to disrupt the normal sequencing of the genes and as such, oncogenes (cancer-promoting genes) on the chromosomes may be "switched on", while tumour suppressors (cancer-preventing genes) may be "switched off".

RISK FACTORS

Numerous risk factors may be associated with DNA damage within the blood cells. Many factors are beyond control (unmodifiable) while others that are environmental and life-style related, are more controllable (modifiable).

The risk factors that are believed to have strong associations with leukemia may include the followings:

- Age.
- Genetics—leukemia risk is increased many-fold amongst people with some genetically linked abnormalities and inherited rare diseases.
- Radiation—the risk of chronic myelogenous leukemia is said to increase with exposure to high doses of radiation. However, it is noted that standard diagnostic x-rays pose little or no increase in leukemia risk.
- Chemicals—the risk for acute leukemia is said to increase many-fold amongst workers with long-term exposure to certain chemicals.
- Viruses.
- Cigarette smoking.
- Cancer therapy—people who have received chemotherapy and radiation therapy for previous cancers have a slightly greater chance of getting secondary leukemia (leukemia that arises after surgery).

TREATMENT

Leukemia is said to involve a number of related cancers that starts in the blood-forming cells of the bone marrow and as such cannot be treated as a single disease. Furthermore, there are both acute and chronic forms of leukemia, each with many sub-types that vary in their response to treatment. Also, children with leukemia have special needs that are best met by care pediatric cancer centres.

The followings are the major approaches to the treatment of leukemia:

- Chemotherapy—to kill off leukemia cells using strong anti-cancer drugs.

- Interferon therapy—to slow the reproduction of leukemia cells and promote the immune system's anti-leukemic activities.

- Radiation therapy—to kill the cancer cells by exposure to high-energy radiation.

- Stem cell transplantation (SCT)—to enable treatment with high doses of chemotherapy and radiation therapy. Stem cells are blood-forming (hematopoietic) cells of the bone marrow; they continuously divide to form new blood cells that populate the arteries and veins. The SCT procedure enables the physician to give chemotherapy and radiotherapy in sufficient doses to eliminate leukemia cells. The injured bone marrow is then replenished by a transplant of stem cells, which can manufacture the necessary new blood cells.

- Surgery—is used to remove an enlarged spleen or to install a venous access device (large plastic tube) to give medication and withdraw blood samples.

The treatment of leukemia is also said to depend on a number of factors. The most important being the histopathologic type of leukemia (disease type); its stage; and certain prognostic factors, such as patient's age and overall health.

Sickle Cell Disease (Anemia)

Sickle cell disease is an inherited blood disorder affecting the haemoglobin in the red blood cells. When blood flows through the lungs, the haemoglobin picks up oxygen. The blood is then pumped by the heart to the body, where the haemoglobin releases the oxygen to the tissues.

Normal red blood cells contain haemoglobin "A", which has a life span of 90-120 days and are then replenished from the bone marrow. Persons with sickle cell disease have mostly haemoglobin "S", which do not live as long as haemoglobin "A"—only about 10-20 days. When red blood cells die, they release their haemoglobin, which the body breaks down and are filtered out by the spleen. The spleen is an organ in the abdomen that filters, removes, and destroys abnormal, damaged, and senile red blood cells and also helps fight infection.

Normal red blood cells have and maintain doughnut-like shape even after releasing their oxygen. When sickle red blood cells give up their oxygen, they become "sickled" or "crescent" shaped. These so-shaped cells do not move easily through the blood vessels and they tend to get stuck and block the flow of blood. When this happens, the blood supply to the organs and tissues is reduced. This causes complications of the sickle cell disease, such as fatigue, breathlessness, rapid heartbeat, susceptibility to infections, vision problems, skin ulcers, and delayed growth.

Sickle cell disease crisis can also be caused by other conditions including a decrease in available oxygen, a viral infection especially involving the lungs, and a state of dehydration. Dehydrated red blood cells are said to rapidly sickle when deoxygenated. Furthermore, sickle red blood cells cannot carry oxygen and they increase the blood viscosity. This can result in lung tissue damage (acute chest syndrome); pain episodes (arms, chest, abdomen, and legs); and stroke. Damage can also be done to most body organs including the kidneys, liver and spleen. This is said to make the sickle cell disease patient easily overwhelmed by certain bacterial infections. Proper personal and medical management can reduce occurrence of crisis.

How does one get sickle cell disease?

Sickle cell disease is a genetic disorder and the only way to get the disease is by genetic inheritance. People with sickle cell disease either have sickle cell trait or sickle cell anemia. The difference between the trait and the disease lies in the inheritance pattern of the sickle cell gene.

Sickle cell condition is inherited from parents in much the same way as blood type, eye colour, hair colour and texture, and other physical traits. The type of haemoglobin the red blood cell makes depend upon what haemoglobin gene is inherited from each parent. Like most genes, haemoglobin genes are inherited in two sets, one from each parent. So it is impossible to acquire sickle cell trait or disease by contact, blood transfusion or any other means.

Unaffected persons have two copies of the haemoglobin "A" (AA). Persons with the trait have one copy each of haemoglobin "A" and haemoglobin "S" (AS). Persons with the disease have two copies of the haemoglobin "S" (SS).

If one parent has sickle anemia (SS) and the other is unaffected (AA), then the children will all have sickle trait (AS). If one parent has sickle anemia (SS) and the other has the trait (AS), then there is 50 per cent chance (1 out of 2) of having an offspring with either sickle cell anemia (SS) or sickle cell trait (AS). There no possibility of having unaffected offspring. If both parents have sickle cell trait, they have a 25 percent chance (1 out of 4) of having offspring with sickle cell anemia. Or it is possible that all children will be unaffected; or all will have the trait; or all will have the disease. If neither parent has the trait, then no children will have the trait or the disease.

People who have inherited two copies of the haemoglobin "S" gene (one from each parent) are homozygous and have sickle cell disease. They cannot make normal haemoglobin "A". Those who have inherited only one copy of the haemoglobin "S" gene have sickle cell trait but also have one copy of haemoglobin "A" and can make normal haemoglobin. People with sickle cell trait usually do not manifest any of the problems associated with sickle cell anemia.

GEOGRAPHIC DISTRIBUTION

The disease is believed to have originated in at least four geographical regions in Africa and the Indian/Saudi Arabian sub-continent. It exists in all countries of Africa and in areas where Africans have migrated.

DIAGNOSIS

Early diagnosis, preferably in the newborn period is advisable. Blood sample is taken for smear test and it can show whether the newborn infant has sickle cell anemia or sickle cell trait. If the first test shows some sickle haemoglobin, then a second is done to confirm the diagnosis.

Haemoglobin (Hgb) Electrophoresis is usually used to confirm the initial result and also to diagnose sickle cell in older children and adults. Electrophoresis is a blood test that looks at how haemoglobin moves in an electric field. Sickle haemoglobin moves differently than normal haemoglobin.

There is also the possibility of identifying sickle cell anemia before birth. This test, which identifies the sickle gene rather than the haemoglobin, is reportedly done using a sample of the amniotic fluid or tissue taken from the placenta. The amniotic fluid is the fluid in the sac surrounding a growing embryo, while the placenta is the organ that attaches the umbilical cord to the mother's womb. The test can be done as early as the first few months of pregnancy.

SIGNS AND SYMPTOMS

The signs and symptoms of sickle cell anemia vary with individuals. Some people have mild symptoms while others have very severe symptoms and are often hospitalised for treatment.

The most common signs and symptoms are linked to anemia and pain crisis while others are linked to some of the complications of the disease.

- Anemia—the general signs and symptoms of anemia are fatigue (tiredness), pale skin, jaundice (yellowing of the skin or whites of the eyes), and shortness of breath.

- Pain crisis—Sudden episodes of pain throughout the body is referred to as sickle cell crisis. A sickle cell crisis occurs when the red blood cells become sickle shaped and then stick together in clumps. These clumps retard the flow of blood through the small blood capillaries in the organs and extremities. Sickle cell crisis can cause acute or chronic pains. Acute pain is said to be sudden and can range from mild to very severe and usually lasts from hours to a few days. Chronic pain usually lasts for weeks to months and can be hard to bear and mentally draining. Many factors can contribute to onset of sickle cell crisis. These can include infection and dehydration. Dehydration is when the body does not have enough fluid. Drinking plenty of fluid often help decrease the chances of a crisis.

- Complications of sickle cell anemia—Complications come from the effect of sickle cell crisis on the different parts of the body such as:—1. Hand/foot crisis—When sickled cells block the small blood vessels in the hands or feet, pain and swelling along with fever can occur. The pain may be felt in the many bones of the hands and feet while swelling usually occurs on the back of the hands and feet and moves into the fingers and toes. One or both hands and/or feet may be affected at the same time. 2. Splenic crisis—Sometimes the spleen traps many sickle cells and grows large and cannot work normally. This causes anemia and blood transfusion may be required until the body can make more blood cells and recover. 3. Infections—Damaged spleen can result in the likelihood of getting infections that can be fatal. Some of the infections can be pneumonia, meningitis, influenza, and hepatitis. 4. Acute chest syndrome—This is characterized by severe chest pain and fever and is caused by sickle cells trapped in the lungs or by associated infections. 5. Pulmonary Artery Hypertension—Damage to the small blood vessels in the lungs can make it hard for the heart to pump blood through the lungs. This causes the blood pressure in the lungs to increase, leading to excessive shortness of breath. 6. Gallstones—When red blood cells die, they release their haemoglobin, which is broken down into a compound called bilirubin. When there is too much of these in the body, stones can be formed in the gallbladder. Gallstones can cause steady pain that can last for thirty minutes or more in the upper right side of the body, under the right shoulder, or between the shoulder blades. 7. Eye problems—When the retina does not get enough blood, it can weaken, causing serious problems, which might include blindness. The retina is a light-sensitive thin layer of tissue at the back of the eye. It takes the images seen and sends them to the brain through the optic nerves. 8. Priapism—Males with sickle cell anemia may have painful and unwanted erections and this happens when the sickle cells stop blood flow out of an erect penis. This is called priapism and can damage the penis and lead to impotence. 9. Stroke—Sickled red blood cells may stick to the walls of the tiny blood vessels in the brain causing a stroke. This type of stroke is said to occur mainly in children and can cause more severe problems.

TREATMENT

Presently, it is reported that there is no cure for sickle cell anemia. But effective treatments are available to help relieve the symptoms and complications of the disease. Some researchers believe bone marrow transplantation may offer a cure in certain cases, and are looking into new treatments such as gene therapy and safer and more effective bone marrow transplants.

Health maintenance for sickle cell disease patients start with early diagnosis and are reported to include penicillin prophylaxis; vaccination against pneumococcus bacteria; and daily folic acid supplementation. Treatment of complications is also said to include antibiotics; pain management with analgesics; intravenous fluids; large regular fluid intake; blood transfusion; and even surgery. All these are backed by psycho-social and family support.

Doctors specializing in the treatment of sickle cell anemia are often haematologists. These are doctors who treat people with blood disorders.

Goal of treatment
The goals of treating sickle cell anemia are to relieve pains; prevent infections, organ damage, and strokes; and control complications if they occur.

Treating pain—Mild painful crisis can be managed with recommended medication and heating pads. However, severe pain may need to be treated in a hospital. Painful crisis are said to be the leading cause of emergency room visits and hospitalizations of people with sickle cell anemia. The usual treatments for acute crisis are pain-killing medications and plenty of fluids, either taken by mouth or given through a vein, to prevent dehydration.

Preventing infections—Opportunistic infection is a major complication of sickle cell anemia. Pneumonia is reported to be a leading cause of death in children with the condition. Other infections said to be common in people with sickle cell anemia include meningitis, influenza, and hepatitis. It is advisable that if a child with sickle cell anemia shows early signs of infection, such as fever, medical treatment should be sort immediately.

To prevent infections, especially in children, recommended treatments may include:—Daily doses of penicillin; daily supplementation of folic acid (to help produce more red blood cells); vaccinations for pneumonia, meningitis, influenza, and hepatitis; and a yearly flu shot.

Preventing eye damage—Sickle cell anemia can damage the blood vessels in the eyes, affecting the retina or causing other problems. It is advisable to consult your doctor about regular checkups with an eye doctor who specializes in diseases of the retina.

Blood transfusions—Blood transfusions are used to treat worsening anemia and sickle cell complications. A sudden worsening case of anemia due to an infection or enlargement of the spleen is a common reason for a blood transfusion. Blood transfusion is also said to help reduce recurrent pain crisis, reduce risk of stroke and other infections. However, not all patients need transfusion since the body can make more and recover during the course of normal treatment.

Regular blood transfusion is said to have side effects. These can include a dangerous buildup of iron in the blood as well as an increased risk of infection from the transfused blood. Red blood cells contain iron, which can accumulate in the blood to a toxic level. There is no natural way for the body to eliminate the excess iron and it may accumulate in the liver and other body organs, leading to damage. Treatments are said to be available to eliminate iron overload. Please discuss with your doctor.

Preventing stroke—Stroke prevention and treatment is possible for people with sickle cell anemia. Regular ultrasound scans of the head are used to monitor the blood flow in the brain. The scans allow the doctors to find out who is at high risk for a stroke and to treat them accordingly.

Treating other complications—Acute chest syndrome is a severe and life-threatening complication in those with sickle cell anemia. Treatment usually requires hospitalization and may include pain medication, antibiotics, oxygen, blood transfusion, monitoring the body's fluid, and ultrasound scan.

Gallbladder surgery may be needed if the presence of gallstones leads to gallbladder disease.

Priapism can be treated with fluids or surgery.

New treatments—Bone marrow transplant procedure is said to be risky and could result in serious side effects and even death. Therefore, it is usually used only for younger patients with severe sickle cell anemia and the decision is only made on individual basis. Bone marrow used for a transplant must come from a closely matched donor, usually a close family member, without sickle cell anemia.

Gene therapy—This is being studied as a possible treatment for sickle cell anemia. Researchers are looking to see if a normal gene can be planted in the bone marrow of a person with sickle cell anemia, and therefore cause the body to produce normal red blood cells. The possibility of treatment to "turn off" the sickle cell gene or "turn on" a gene that makes normal red blood cells is also being studied.

Please continually discuss developments in treatment and therapy with your doctor or healthcare worker.

Living with sickle cell disease

Sickle cell trait (AS) is an inherited condition in which both haemoglobin "A" and "S" are produced in the red blood cells but always more "A" than "S". Sickle cell trait is not a type of sickle cell disease and people with sickle cell trait are generally healthy. People with sickle cell anemia (SS) have inherited two copies of the haemoglobin "S" and cannot make normal haemoglobin "A" in their red blood cells. They exhibit all the complications of the disease. However, this is not a death sentence. With proper healthcare maintenance and psycho-social support, some live a normal life—no sicker than someone with normal haemoglobin "A" in their red blood cells.

People of African origin or from susceptible geographical regions should be tested and know their blood genotypes. Early diagnosis, preferably in the newborn period is advisable.

Those with sickle cell trait (AS) that wishes to get married or become pregnant are advised to get genetic counselling to determine their risk of having offsprings with the trait or the disease.

Some other factors that reportedly modify the severity of sickle cell disease are the halotypes of the betaglobin gene cluster and foetal haemoglobin (Hbf) expression. The Senegal halotype is associated with the most benign form of sickle cell disease, followed by the Benin halotype while the Central African Republic halotype is associated with the most severe form of the disease. Some treatments such as penicillin prophylaxis and hydroxyurea have been reportedly developed and targeted at raising the levels of the foetal haemoglobin (Hbf) and said to significantly reduce the morbidity and mortality of sickle cell disease.

Individuals with sickle cell trait (AS) are reported to have decreased risk of infection by the malaria parasite (plasmodium falciparum). However, malaria is fatal in those with the disease (SS), and therefore should be protected against malaria infection. Sleeping under the protection of insecticide-treated mosquito net and regular anti-malarial drug administration are recommended.

Hydroxyurea is reported may be given daily to young adolescents and adults with severe sickle cell anemia to reduce their number of painful crisis and acute chest syndrome. This drug is said to be used for crisis prevention only and not for treatment when they occur. There is also the risk of reported side effects, which should be discussed with your doctor.

Good personal hygiene to reduce the risk of opportunistic bacterial infection; and avoidance of extreme physical stress or low atmospheric oxygen can reduce the on-set of sickle cell anemia crisis. With good healthcare, many people with sickle cell anemia can live productive lives, with good health much of the time, and live longer today than in the past. Many people with sickle cell anemia now live into their forties or fifties, or longer.

To take care of your health, it is important to maintain healthy lifestyle habits, do what you can to prevent onset of sickle cell crisis, get regular medical care, and learn what signs to watch out for. Some of these should include:

- Eating healthy and the doctor may also recommend daily supplementation of folic acid to help your body make new red blood cells.

- Drinking plenty of water (at least eight glasses) daily, especially in warm weather to prevent dehydration.

- Getting enough sleep and rest.

- Limiting the amount of alcohol you drink.

- Quitting smoking, if you smoke.

- Avoid extremes of heat and cold. Wear warm clothes outside in cold weather and inside of air-conditioned rooms. Do not swim in cold water.

- Avoid climbing at high altitudes without extra oxygen and avoid travelling in unpressurized cabin airplanes. If you must travel in such airplanes, talk to your doctor and airline staff about how to protect yourself.

- Reduce stress in your life. Talk to your doctor if you are depressed or having problems on the job or with your personal life. If possible do not seek jobs that will require strenuous physical labour, expose you to extremes of heat and cold, or involve long work hours.

- Contact your doctor if you have any signs of an infection, such as a fever or trouble breathing

- Visit a doctor (haematologist) regularly and checkups may include tests for any kidney, lungs, and liver diseases as well as side effects from regular medications.

- Learn stroke symptoms and report any promptly to your doctor.

- Get the recommended vaccinations and a flu shot to prevent infections.

- Visit an eye doctor regularly to check for any eye damage and get treatment and control any other medical condition you might have, such as diabetes.

- As a lady, talk to your doctor if you are pregnant or planning to become pregnant. Special prenatal care will be needed. Sickle cell anemia can become more severe during pregnancy, with more crisis, but you can have a normal pregnancy with early prenatal care and frequent checkups.

Coping with pain—Pains and pain tolerance are different with individuals. Work out with your doctor to make a pain management plan that works well for you. It may include over-the-counter or prescription medication. Other ways to manage pain may include using heating pad, taking a hot bath, resting, or getting a massage. Physical therapy that can help relax and strengthen the muscles and joints may be helpful. Also helpful are activities that can keep your mind off the pain, such as watching TV and talking with friends.

Caring for a child with sickle cell anemia—Although sickle cell anemia is present at birth, many infants do not show any signs until about four months of age. Parents should learn as much about the condition as possible. This will help to recognize early signs of problems, such as fever or chest pain, and seek early treatment. The first sign of sickle cell anemia in infants may be pains (felt in the many bones of the hands and feet) and swelling (usually at the back of the hands and feet, moving into the fingers and toes). This is hand-foot syndrome. Sickle cell centres and clinics usually give information and counselling that can help you handle the stresses of coping with this serious and chronic condition.

It is advisable to talk to your child's doctor about the child's treatment, frequency of visits, what to report right away, and the best ways of keeping the child as healthy as possible. You may need to call the doctor immediately if the child has a fever, or has any signs of an infection or stroke. It is advisable to keep a thermometer and know how to use it, and also know the signs and symptoms of a possible stroke.

Ask the child's doctor of the requirement for regular ultrasound scans of the head to assess the risk of a stroke and need for early treatment.

School-aged children may participate in physical education and sports, but only after approval of the child's doctor and with regular checks. Ask the doctor about safe levels of exercise for the child.

Caring for a teen with sickle cell anemia—Teens with sickle cell anemia must manage their condition while dealing with other stresses of teen years. These may include peer pressure, sexuality, education, independence, and career goals. Specific stresses faced by teens with sickle cell anemia is said to include some of the followings:

- Body-image problems caused by a delayed growth or sexual maturity.
- Coping with pain and fear of addiction and side effects of pain and regular medications.
- Living with uncertainty, because the disease is unpredictable and can cause pain and damage to the body at any time.

The ways to support teens with sickle cell anemia include teen support groups and family and individual counselling.

Experience of someone with sickle cell anemia

This is an adult with sickle cell anemia and has been living a normal life, no sicker than any other adult. He has had sickle cell crisis only once in early childhood that resulted in hospital stay and a blood transfusion.

Sometime ago, the patient came down with high body temperature and abdominal pains and was diagnosed with urinary tracts infection (UTI). He was treated with antibiotics (ciprofloxacin) twice daily for about five days and felt better after the course of the treatment. A week later, he was back on admission in hospital with chronic abdominal and chest pain. Suspicion was that the infection was back and may have affected other body organs such as the kidneys or heart.

He was setup with continuous intravenous drip, with administration of analgesic (for pain relief) and antibiotics (for combating the infections). Treatment also included daily folic acid supplementation with enough oral fluid (water) intakes to prevent dehydration and ensure normal blood viscosity.

Various diagnostic tests were carried out including CT scan, ECG, ultrasound test, lateral lung scan, and regular (daily) blood tests. The battery of tests was to confirm, manage, or monitor the infections in the organs and the blood tests to check progression or remission of the infections. Blood haemoglobin levels were also constantly monitored. Blood thinning medication was injected through the stomach muscle to help reduce blood viscosity and improve circulation, thereby relieving crisis level due to sickling of the red blood cells haemoglobin.

This is a case of opportunistic infection precipitating a chronic sickle cell crisis. During the course of the treatment when the haemoglobin level dropped to about 5.9g/dl, blood transfusion was considered but the haemoglobin level gradually crept up to 6.2g/dl and stabilised. The blood transfusion was aborted as the body was fighting the infection and responding to the treatment regimes.

The chest pain (chest syndrome), abdominal pain and high body temperature gradually abated with continued treatment. Generous fluid intake continued both orally and intravenous.

After about two week's hospitalisation, he was discharged from the haematological department and placed on daily dosage of folic acid and penicillin VK 250mg. He was also recommended for the following vaccines—pneomorax, HIB, and menintococcus.

He is fully recovered and living a normal life.

What is a risk factor or risk profile?

A risk factor can be described as anything that may increase a person's chance of developing a certain disease. Although these factors can increase a person's risk, they may not necessarily cause the disease and someone with one or more risk factors may never develop the disease, while others with no known risk factors, may develop it.

Risk factors may include family history, cholesterol and triglycerides level, congenital disorders, diet, blood pressure, smoking, weight, stress level and many other things. Different diseases have different risk factors and knowing one's risk factors to any disease can help guide to appropriate actions, including behavioural and lifestyle changes and being clinically monitored for the disease.

Risk factors can be labelled as controllable (modifiable) or uncontrollable (unmodifiable). The uncontrollable risk factors may include age, gender, family history of the disease or congenital (present at birth) conditions.

Blood Pressure

Blood pressure is the force created by the heart contracting to keep the blood circulating adequately and constantly through the blood vessels of the body. In order to overcome the resistance that is present in miles of narrow blood vessels and in order for the blood to finally arrive at the tissues with enough residual pressure to affect an interchange of chemicals, the heart must maintain a certain minimal level of pressure within the circulatory system.

Blood pressure is measured using two values, say, a blood pressure of 120 over 80, written as 120/80mm Hg. Both pressures are recorded as "mm Hg" (millimetres of mercury) and represents how high the column of mercury is raised by the pressure of blood. The first figure is the maximum pressure in the arteries when the heart contracts and pumps blood out into the body (active or systolic pressure). The second figure is the minimum pressure in the arteries between beats when the heart relaxes to fill with blood (restive or diastolic pressure). There is a wide range of pressures considered normal for the average adult and an average reading might be 120/80 millimetres of mercury. The upper limit of normal systolic pressure is said to be about 150-160mm of mercury, and the upper limit of the diastolic pressure is from 90-100mm of mercury.

Blood pressure rises naturally with age due to the reduced elasticity of the arterial system and also varies with time of day and other variables. So, an isolated high reading may not mean much. If high blood pressure is suspected, the doctor will have the patient in for several times of repeated measurements for confirmation.

Blood Pressure Reading

Blood Pressure Reading—Blood pressure is measured using adapted manual or digital pressure monitoring instrument. A tubular rubber cuff is strapped around the upper arm. The cuff is connected to an apparatus that measures pressure, and it is inflated with air while the physician listens to the arterial pulse in the crock of the elbow with a stethoscope. The air pressure in the cuff is raised until the pulsation can no longer be heard. After this, the cuff is deflated until the pulse beat returns; this point is noted as the systolic pressure. The cuff is further gradually deflated until the pulse beat again disappears; the pressure at this point is called the diastolic pressure. Different types of digital blood pressure readers are available, using the same principles but with the readings digitally displayed. Some models also display the heart beat rate with data storage memory.

High Blood Pressure

Blood pressure depends on a combination of how forcefully the heart pumps blood and how narrowed or relaxed the arteries are. High blood pressure or Hypertension occurs when blood is forced through the arteries at an increased pressure.

It is believed that narrowing of the arteries throughout the body causes the heart to pump harder to get blood through to the various tissues. When the heart pumps harder, blood pressure is elevated. Thus; greater than average strain is placed upon the heart and if prolonged, the heart may become enlarged and damaged. Also, greater wear and tear is placed upon all the blood vessels; since blood flows through them at greater pressure and eventually, severe damage maybe inflicted upon the vessels. This in turn may cause impairment of function of the tissues and organs that the vessels supply.

High blood pressure rarely causes symptoms, so it might go unnoticed until it causes later complications such as: stroke, heart attack, atherosclerosis, heart failure (reduced pumping ability), kidney failure and eye damage. Also, severe hypertension may cause symptoms such as headache, sleepiness, confusion and eventually coma.

RISK FACTORS

Risk Factors:—Certain factors are said to initiate or aggravate hypertension and increase the risk of complications. These factors include:—

- Tendency for hypertension to run in the family (familial tendency).
- Obesity.
- Diabetes.
- Arteriosclerosis (hardening and narrowing of the arteries).
- High blood cholesterol level (LDL).

- Kidney disease.
- High alcohol intake.
- Smoking.
- Excessive salt intake.
- Lack of exercise.
- Hormonal disturbances.
- Drug (steroids) abuse.

All these can result in "secondary hypertension" while "primary or essential hypertension" is still thought to be of unknown cause.

Doctors can assess risk factors and help initiate lifestyle changes to reduce the risks or lower the already high blood pressure. Some of these recommended actions might include:—1. To stop smoking. 2 Loose weight, if over weight. 3. Cutting down on alcohol. 4. Regular exercise. 5. Reduce stress by avoiding stressful situations or by trying different relaxation techniques. 6. Eating a balanced (varied), low-fat, low-salt diet. 7. Reduce blood cholesterol level (LDL).

Medication may also be offered for reduction of high blood pressure. Regular monitoring is required to ensure that the blood pressure is under good control.

Arteriosclerosis

This is the hardening and narrowing of the blood arteries, resulting from plaque build-up in the arterial walls. The normal walls of an artery is strong, supple and elastic so that it can expand and contract in adjustment to the changes in blood pressure, which takes place with heart contraction. But when an artery becomes hardened or atherosclerotic, its walls are rigid and pipe-like instead of elastic. This can be caused by abnormal deposits within the walls of the artery that causes gradual narrowing and may eventually seal the vessel completely so that no blood can flow through it.

The exact trigger is unverified but current research is said to indicate that wear and tear upon the blood vessels and faulty metabolism of fatty substances such as cholesterol produces arteriosclerosis. As the blood vessels are damaged, patches of cholesterol are deposited at the site in repair attempt; thus building up more plaque.

RISK FACTORS

Risk Factors:—Arteriosclerosis is said to affect lots of people, even in their teens and increases with age. It is a slow, progressive disease that may start as early as childhood and has the potential to progress rapidly. Although the exact cause is unknown, several risk factors have been identified that accelerate the disease. These factors include:—1. Family history of the disease. 2. Hypertension (high blood pressure). 3. High blood cholesterol. 4. Diabetes. 5. Excessive weight. 6. Smoking. 7. Stress. 8. Lack of exercise. 9. Unhealthy diet.

Symptoms of arteriosclerosis depend on the body part that the affected blood artery supplies:—In the brain (cerebrovascular disease), the presence of arterial plaque can lead to a blood clot (thrombus); thus cutting off oxygen supply to the brain area or the affected artery may also rupture (haemorrhage) and cause considerable brain damage. Both incidents are known as stroke (cerebrovascular accidents or CVAs). Stroke normally produces a sudden onset of symptoms such as paralysis, visual and sensory disturbances, speech and swallowing difficulties-depending on the affected artery.

In the heart (cardiovascular disease); it can manifest as angina, coronary thrombosis or heart failure (reduced heart efficiency) due to damage done to the heart muscle.

In the kidney, it can lead to high blood pressure and renal failure.

In the legs (peripheral vascular disease); cramping pain can be experienced due to hardening in the main and smaller arteries to the lower limbs and in extreme cases amputation of the leg due to restricted blood supply.

It is reported that there is currently no medication available to cure arteriosclerosis or drugs to make diseased arteries regain their elasticity. However, changes in lifestyle, medication and cholesterol-lowering regime can reduce the risk factors, retard progression of the disease and the likelihood of plaque rupture. Also, medication to prevent blood clotting (thrombosis) may be recommended. If the risk factors can be minimised then the development of the disease can be slowed down.

Vascular disease is a manifestation of arteriosclerosis which has developed over a period of time, and can result in disability or premature death if unspotted and progression unchecked. Heart attack (coronary thrombosis) and stroke (cerebrovascular accident) are reportedly the commonest causes of premature deaths. Please seek medical advice if you discover symptoms suggestive of vascular disease or at risk of the disease.

Thrombosis

Blood vessel thrombosis is the formation of a blood clot within the vessel, in either an artery or a vein. Veins are blood vessels that carry blood from the body back to the heart, while arteries are the blood vessels that carry oxygenated blood away from the heart to the body. Venous thrombosis is when the blood clot obstructs a vein, and arterial thrombosis is when the blood clot obstructs an artery.

CAUSES

Causes:—Arterial thrombosis is said to be result of atherosclerosis (hardening of the arteries) of the blood vessels. When arterial thrombosis occurs in the coronary arteries, it may lead to heart attacks. When it occurs in the cerebral or brain circulation, it can lead to strokes or lack of oxygen to other organs.

Venous thrombosis may be caused by the following:

- Inherited disorders or predisposition to thrombosis. Congenital or acquired blood coagulation protein or platelet defect is said to cause or contribute to the thrombotic event.
- Disease or injury to the veins in the legs (deep veins).
- Immobility
- Bone fractures.
- Obesity.
- Certain medications.

Symptoms

Symptoms:—Pooling of blood in the legs due to inactivity and subsequent clotting can result in varicose veins. The clotting may break loose and travel to the lungs, causing pulmonary clots that can result in respiratory distress, pain, and maybe death.

Each individual may experience thrombotic symptoms differently, but some of these symptoms may include:

- Varicose veins.
- Swelling in the extremities.
- Isolated leg pains, usually the calf or thigh muscles.
- Increased blood clots in the arteries or veins.

These symptoms are not exclusively for thrombosis and may resemble other blood disorders or medical problems. Please always consult your doctor for diagnosis of symptoms and treatment.

Treatment

Treatment:—Specific treatment for thrombosis will be determined by the doctor based on age; overall health; medical history; extent and type of thrombosis; and tolerance for specific medications, procedures, or therapies. Treatment may also include anticoagulant and clot dissolving medications, and catheters to expand the width of the involved blood vessels.

Embolism

Embolism is said to be an obstruction in a blood vessel due to either a blood clot or other foreign matter that gets stuck while travelling through the bloodstream. The emboli (plural of embolus) are usually formed from blood clots but are occasionally comprised of air, fat, or tumour tissue. There are three general categories of emboli: arterial, gas, and pulmonary. Pulmonary emboli are reportedly the most common. Embolic events can be small and multiple, or single and massive.

Arterial embolism:—This is generally a complication of heart disease, where blood flow is blocked at the junction of major arteries, most often at the groin, knee, or thigh. An arterial embolism in the brain (cerebral embolism) causes stroke. Arterial emboli to the extremities can lead to tissue death and amputation of the affected limb. Kidneys and intestines can also suffer damage from emboli.

Gas embolism:—This can result from the compression of respiratory gases into the blood and other tissues due to rapid changes in environmental pressure, as in, while flying or scuba diving. During scuba diving, the body is deep under water and it is subjected to strong pressures; therefore certain gases (nitrogen) are absorbed into the blood. As external pressure decreases, (by returning to the surface from water depth or flying in an airplane at high cabin altitudes), gases (nitrogen) that are dissolved in the blood and other tissues become small bubbles that can block blood flow or cause severe pains and organ damage. Gas bubbles in the blood is also said to cause great pain and some immobilisation in the shoulders, arms, and joints. This complaint is called decompression sickness or the bends.

Pulmonary embolism:—This is caused by blood clots that travel through the blood stream to the lungs and block a pulmonary artery. A high percentage of cases of pulmonary embolism are reported to be complications of deep vein thrombosis, which may typically occur in patients with cancer or who have had orthopaedic surgery, and also patients with other related illnesses like congestive heart failure.

RISK FACTORS

Risk factors for gas emboli are reported to include:

- Scuba diving-especially before flying. Scuba diving and flying do not mix. As a guide, it is advisable not to fly within twelve hours of any scuba diving.
- Amateur flight manoeuvres.
- Some exercises.
- Obesity.
- Injury.
- Excessive alcohol intake.
- Dehydration.
- Some medications such as narcotics and antihistamines.

Risk factors for pulmonary and arterial emboli are reported to include:

- Heart attack and congestive heart failure.
- Stroke.
- Surgery and a broken hip or leg.
- Sickle cell anemia and chest trauma.
- Some congenital heart defects.
- Sedentary live or prolonged bed rest.
- Obesity.
- Some oral contraceptive and child birth.

SYMPTOMS

Some symptoms of pulmonary embolism may include: a rapid or laboured breathing, sometimes accompanied by chest pain; a cough that may produce bloodied sputum; fluid build-up in the lungs; leg swelling; swollen neck veins; and pain caused by movement or breathing.

Some symptoms of arterial embolism is said to include: tingling or severe pain in the area of the embolism; numbness or muscular weakness or paralysis.

The listed symptoms are not solely for embolism and can be indicative of other medical conditions and it is therefore important to consult your doctor for diagnosis and treatment. An embolism can be diagnosed by the physician through the patient's medical history, physical examination, and diagnostic tests. Some of these tests might include: For pulmonary embolism: chest x-ray, lung scan, electrocardiography (ECG), pulmonary angiography, venography or venous ultrasound, and arterial blood gas measurement. And for arterial embolism: cardiac ultrasound and/or arteriography.

Deep Vein Thrombosis (DVT)

Thrombosis is said to occur when the blood changes from its liquid form to a jelly-like state, producing a clot. If the blood clot occurs within a major vein, then the condition is known as deep vein thrombosis. The most commonly affected veins by DVT are the deep veins of the lower leg (calf) and thigh, up to the pelvic region. Rarely, it can develop in other deep veins, say, in the arm. It is possible to have a small DVT without being aware of it; but the condition only becomes dangerous or possibly fatal, if the blood clot is big enough to cause an occlusion (blockage).

The large deep veins of the legs and pelvic region can form clots of considerable size that becomes potentially hazardous if they move. Such clots can form during long periods of inactivity; and when there is sudden movement, blood flow will increase within the veins and the clot or part thereof can break-off. This clot can travel upwards toward the heart and may end up in the lungs (pulmonary embolism); eventually causing death. The blood clot can also either partially or completely block the flow of blood in the vein.

Symptoms and Complications

Many blood clots occurring in DVT are said to be small and may not cause any symptoms; and the body will eventually be able to break them down with no long-term effects. Large clots may block the blood flow in the vein and cause the following symptoms:

- Swelling of the affected leg (usually different from mild swelling of both ankles associated with long-haul flights, due to lack of muscle movement that helps drain away tissue fluid)

- Localised pain or tenderness within the affected leg muscles—becoming noticeable or worse when standing or walking.

- Reddening of the affected leg.

Although it may not necessarily be as a result of DVT, if any of the symptoms is experienced, it is advisable to consult a medical practitioner immediately.

Possible complications of DVT may include the followings:

Pulmonary embolism—this happens when a piece of the blood clot from a DVT breaks off and travels through the bloodstream to the lungs. In the lungs it can block a pulmonary artery. This can cause chest pain or palpitations, breathlessness, increased heart rate or sudden onset of coughing; and may be fatal. Pulmonary embolism (PE) can happen hours or even days after the DVT has formed, and may occur without any obvious signs of a DVT. Please seek emergency medical treatment for any symptom of PE.

Post-thrombotic syndrome—this is said to happen if DVT damages the valves in the deep veins, so that instead of flowing upwards, the blood pools in the lower leg. This can eventually lead to long-term pain, swelling and in severe cases, ulcers in the leg.

Limb ischaemia—this is a rear complication that only happens in severe DVT. Due to blood clot in the leg vein, the pressure in the vein can become very high. This can reduce the blood flow through the arteries, so less oxygen and nutrients is carried to the affected leg.

OTHER RISK FACTORS

There are a number of other reported risk factors that may increase the chances of developing DVT—these include:

- Inherited blood clotting disorders.
- Medical blood clotting diseases.
- Being over 40 years old.
- Being over weight.
- Having had DVT before.
- Having had recent surgery or injury—especially to the hips or knees.
- Being a smoker.
- Certain blood diseases.

- Circulation problems or heart failure.

- Cancer or have had cancer treatment.

- Being on the pills (ladies).

- Taking hormone replacement therapy (HRT) (ladies).

- Being pregnant or having recently had a baby (ladies).

TRAVEL RISKS (LONG-HAUL FLIGHTS)

DVT maybe associated with any form of long distance travel whether by air, car, coach or train as this journey can lead to increase in the risk of blood clots forming in the veins of the legs.

There is suggestive evidence however, that long-haul flights (flight lasting four hours or more) may increase the risk of developing DVT. This risk is said to be mainly due to prolonged immobility and dehydration associated with high altitude flights.

Most modern passenger aircrafts fly at high altitudes for efficient and economical operations.

Air is a mixture of various gases that are held close to the earth by the force of gravity and because air is compressible, it is "thicker" around the earth's surface. The air density decreases with altitude. The main air components are oxygen (twenty-one percent), nitrogen (seventy-eight percent), and other gases (one percent).

Low air density at high altitude is beneficial to aircraft performance but would expose the occupants to oxygen deficiency and low ambient temperatures. Therefore, the crew and passengers need to be comfortable without the use of oxygen masks and protective body suits. This comfortable environment is provided by maintaining the aircraft cabin environment close to that obtainable at lower altitude; with denser air (more oxygen) and warmer temperature. And to achieve this, compressed air is bled from the aircraft engines; and through a system of filtration, conditioning and regulation, it is used to pressurise the aircraft cabin to a comfortable environment.

Due to pressurization, the aircraft cabin can become very dry with the likelihood of passengers becoming dehydrated. With dehydration, the blood is said to become thicker than usual and therefore more prone to clotting. Moreover, most air travellers do not drink enough fluid when flying and consumes readily available alcoholic drinks, which then makes them use the toilet more. So, unless enough non-alcoholic fluid is taken to compensate, this increases dehydration.

Also, due to limited movement opportunities on board airplanes, blood circulation becomes sluggish. Cramped seating may also cause pressure points on the lower limb that slows down local blood flow, resulting in the possibility of clot formation.

Generally, the risk of developing DVT when travelling is said to be small unless there are other risk factors present. There may be other unresolved factors involved because DVT has also been observed amongst business and first class passengers with more leg room and also equally observed in other types of long journeys.

Simple in-flight exercises and getting up and walking around regularly are advised.

One should seek urgent medical advice if swelling or pain develops in the calf or thigh muscle, or if breathing problems or chest pain is experienced after travelling.

TREATMENT

Because DVT can occur with little or no warning, it is best to adopt preventive actions, which might include reducing manageable risk factors. If DVT symptoms are being experienced, then it is advisable to consult the doctor immediately. And if DVT is diagnosed, the doctor will take the patient's medical history, carry out medical examinations and may recommend further tests. The treatments that may alleviate the effects may include medications and surgical procedures. Practical measures to minimise pain and discomfort may be recommended and may include:—Elevating the affected leg whenever possible; applying heat to relieve pain and reduce swelling; wearing compression bandages or support hose; and avoiding long periods of immobility.

CAUTIONS DURING LONG JOURNEYS

To reduce the added risk of developing DVT on long journeys, there are some preventive measures that can be taken. These may include the followings:

- Be comfortable in your seat.

- Wear loose-fitting clothes.
- Keep hydrated by drinking enough water.
- Avoid excessive alcohol or caffeinated drinks that might increase dehydration.
- Avoid taking sleeping pills, which might also cause immobility.
- Take off shoes to prevent swelling up of feet or wear expandable shoes.
- Take short walks along the aisle when safe to do so.
- Exercise the muscles of the lower legs, which act as a pump for the blood in the veins—regularly bend and straighten your toes, ankles and legs.
- Pressing the balls of your feet down hard against the floor or footrest will also help increase the blood flow in your legs and reduce clotting.
- Upper body and breathing exercises can further improve circulation.
- Try to touch your toes when waiting in the aisle to stretch your hamstrings.
- Wear graduated compression stockings if you have other risk factors for DVT.

It is advisable to seek urgent medical advice if one develops pain or swelling in the calf or thigh muscles, or have breathing problems or chest pain after travelling.

Part Two:

The Heart

Heart

The heart is the motor or main source of energy, which supplies the propelling force to keep the blood stream in motion through all blood vessels of the body. The heart is, in the simplest form, a pump made up of muscle tissue (myocardium) and requires a source of energy and oxygen in order to operate. The heart's pumping action is said to come from an intrinsic electrical conduction system within the heart. This organ, hardly larger than a fist, pumps an average of about 1500gals (6000quarts) of blood daily and this can be increased when necessary.

The heart consists of four chambers; two upper chambers (atria) and two lower chambers (ventricles). There are four one-way heart valves, which direct blood flow into and out of the chambers and between the chambers. The muscle fibres of the heart's chambers is said to contract and relax at timed intervals, creating a pulse and forcing blood through the one-way heart valves; and moving it through the network of arteries.

The heart beats incessantly during life, contracting at an average rate of seventy-eight times per minute, or approximately a hundred and ten thousand times daily to pump blood around the body. Because of this de-fatigability, the thick heart muscles require coronary blood vessels to deliver blood deep into it. Coronary arteries are the blood vessels that spread throughout the walls of the heart, nourishing the heart muscles. The coronary arteries deliver oxygen-rich blood to the heart muscle, while the cardiac veins remove the de-oxygenated blood. The coronary arteries that run on the surface of the heart are said to be capable of auto regulation; to maintain coronary blood flow at levels appropriate to the needs of the heart muscle. These arteries are also known as epicardial arteries and the arteries that run deep within the myocardium are called subendocardial arteries. The coronary arteries are the only source of blood supply to the heart muscle with very little redundancy, and that is why any blockage of these vessels can be critical.

Poor heart action can lead to poor circulation, which in turn leads to derangement and impairment of the function of the vital tissues of the body.

Heart Valves

What are heart valves?

The heart is composed of four compartments. It is divided into a left and a right side, each of which has two connecting chambers—an atrium and a ventricle. Between the chambers are the heart valves. The valves prevent backward flow of blood. These valves are flaps that are located on each end of the two ventricles (lower heart chambers). They act as one-way inlets of blood on one side of a ventricle and one-way outlets of blood on the other side of a ventricle.

The four heart valves include the following:

- Tricuspid valve; located between the right atrium and the right ventricle.
- Pulmonary valve; located between the right ventricle and the pulmonary artery.
- Mitral valve; located between the left atrium and the left ventricle.
- Aortic valve; located between the left ventricle and the aorta.

Normal valves have three flaps, except the mitral valve, which has two flaps.

How the heart valves function

As the heart muscle contracts and relaxes, the valves opens and shut, letting blood flow into the ventricles and atria at alternate times. The right atrium receives blood from all the veins of the body through the two big veins, the inferior and superior veins (vena cavas). This blood is dark red in colour; having a high proportion of waste carbon dioxide and other waste products absorbed from the intestinal tract or released by the tissues. From the right atrium, this blood is directed through the tricuspid valve into the right ventricle. From there, the blood passes through another heart valve—the pulmonic valve and then enters the blood vessels of the lungs. Here, the oxygen supply of the venous blood is replenished and the waste carbon dioxide is exhaled out.

From the lungs, the re-oxygenated blood passes on to the left side of the heart, entering the left atrium. From here it passes through an intervening valve—the mitral valve, and is directed into the powerful and muscular left ventricle. The left ventricle expels the oxygenated blood through the aortic valve into the largest artery of the body—the aorta. From thereon the blood is distributed to all the blood vessels and body tissues.

The unidirectional valves actually channel the flow of blood correctly through the heart chambers.

Heart valve disease

Heart valves malfunction can be sub-divided into two categories. These are:

- Narrowed valves (stenosis). The valves opening become narrowed or the valves become damaged or scarred, inhibiting the flow of blood out of the ventricles or atria. The heart is then forced to pump harder in order to move blood through the damaged valves.
- Leaking valves (regurgitation). The valves do not close completely, causing the blood to flow backward instead of forward through the valves.

Heart valves can have both malfunctions at the same time and more than one valve can also be affected at the same time. When heart valves fail to open or close properly, the implications for the heart can be very serious, possibly hampering the heart's ability to pump blood efficiently. Heart valve problems can eventually result in heart failure.

CAUSES

Causes:—Narrowed valves (stenosis) may be due to:-

- Degeneration through atherosclerosis.
- Damage from rheumatic fever.
- Excessive calcification—in old age.
- Congenital abnormality.

Leaking valves (regurgitation) may be due to:-

- Bacterial infection.
- Valve inflammation.
- Excessive floppiness of the valve leaflets (valve prolapse).

- Enlargement of the heart.
- Enlargement of the aorta.

SYMPTOMS

Failure in a valve in the left side of the heart—the aortic or the mitral valve, results in left-sided failure. This can lead to an accumulation of fluid in the lungs (pulmonary oedema).

Valve diseases of the right side of the heart—the pulmonary or tricuspid valve are uncommon but can occur as a result of some forms of congenital heart disease or long-term left-sided heart failure. Right-sided heart failure can be characterized by fluid accumulation in the body, especially the legs, abdominal cavity and the liver.

Mild cases of heart valve disease may show no symptoms and can be self recovery. More severe cases can manifest some of the reported symptoms. However, some serious cases may also be banal for a long time even though the heart is already under strain.

Some cases of heart valve disease such as narrowed aortic valve (stenosis of the aortic valve), might show symptoms such as:

- Dizziness or faint brought on by physical excersion.
- Shortness of breath.
- Chest pain (angina) on excersion.

A serious untreated heart valve malfunction can lead to heart failure and may eventually result in death.

Antibiotics treatment might be recommended to reduce heart valve infections risk during some medical processes such as; surgical procedures, cardiac catheterisation or dental procedures, where there might be a chance of temporary introduction of some bacteria into the blood stream.

It is important to be aware of the symptoms of the disease and advisable to contact your doctor if any symptom is experienced or even suspected.

Rheumatic heart disease/ rheumatic fever

Rheumatic heart disease is a condition in which permanent damage to the heart valves is caused by rheumatic fever. The heart valve can be damaged by a disease process that generally begins with a "strep throat" caused by streptococcus "A" bacteria, which may eventually cause rheumatic fever. Rheumatic fever is said to usually occur in children—five to fifteen years old, but can also occur at any age.

Rheumatic fever causes heart damage; particularly scarring of the heart valves—forcing the heart to work harder to pump blood and may eventually cause congestive heart failure. It is also an inflammatory disease and can affect many connective tissues, especially in the heart, joints, skin or brain.

SYMPTOMS OF RHEUMATIC FEVER

Symptoms may vary differently with individuals and it typically begins one to six weeks after a bout of "strep throat", although, in some cases, the infection may have been too mild to have been recognized. Symptoms may include:

- Fever.
- Nodules over swollen joints.
- Swollen, tender, red and extremely painful joints—particularly the knees, ankles, elbows or wrists.
- Red, raised, lattice-like rash, usually on the chest, back, or abdomen.
- Uncontrolled spasm of the arms, legs, or facial muscles.
- Weakness and shortness of breath.

The symptoms of rheumatic fever may resemble other disorders or medical conditions. It is therefore, advisable to consult your doctor for a diagnosis.

TREATMENT FOR RHEUMATIC HEART DISEASE

Treatment for rheumatic heart disease will be determined by the physician based on the patient's medical history; overall health; extent of the disease; and tolerance for specific medications, procedures or therapies.

Since rheumatic fever is the cause of rheumatic heart disease, the best treatment is to prevent rheumatic fever from occurring. It is said that penicillin and other antibiotics can usually treat "strep throat" (a streptococcus "A" bacterial infection) and stop acute rheumatic fever from developing.

Persons who have previously had rheumatic fever are often given continuous (daily or monthly) antibiotic treatment to prevent future attacks of rheumatic fever and lower the risk of heart damage. To reduce inflammation, aspirin, steroids, or non-steroidal medications may be given. Surgery may be necessary to repair or replace damaged heart valve.

Your physician will determine the appropriate course of treatment.

Part Three:

Cardiovascular and Coronary Artery Diseases

Cardiovascular Disease (CVD)

The cardiovascular or circulatory system moves blood around the body, carrying oxygen and nutrients to the body tissues and removing waste products such as carbon dioxide and cell waste. Cardiovascular disease encompasses all diseases of the heart and surrounding blood vessels and it is reported to account for more deaths than any other disease worldwide. Heart disease is a general term referring to a variety of medical conditions affecting the heart including heart attack, congenial heart failure and angina.

Heart failure, also medically known as cardiac decompensation, is when the heart is no longer able to accommodate the normal circulatory requirements of the body. Normally, the heart has sufficient reserve strength to compensate for most ordinary handicaps in some disorders, however, as the disorder increases in severity and as the heart muscle becomes more and more fatigued, the heart becomes increasingly incapable of meeting its obligation.

Heart attack occurs when the blood supply to part of the heart muscle is reduced or stops due to a blockage in one or more of the heart's arteries (coronary arteries).

Stroke affects the arteries leading to and from the brain and can be caused by either a blockage or rupture reducing blood flow and thus preventing vital oxygen and nutrients reaching the brain; starving cells and causing potentially irreparable damage.

Angina is a cardiovascular disease of pain in the chest area often brought on by excersion.

Coronary artery disease

Coronary artery disease (CAD) is characterised by the accumulation of plaque and fatty deposits inside the coronary arteries. These deposits may start early and continue to thicken and enlarge throughout life span and narrows the arteries. This can decrease or block the flow of blood to the heart.

Coronary arteries are the blood vessels that spread throughout the walls of the heart, supplying the heart muscles with blood and nourishing it. These are the first blood vessels to branch off the aorta (the main artery from the left ventricle of the heart) as it leaves the heart.

The symptoms of coronary heart disease depend on its severity. If less oxygenated blood reaches the heart, chest pain or angina will be experienced. When the blood supply is completely cut off, the result is said to be a heart attack, and the heart muscle then begins to die. A heart attack is said to be "silent" when the symptoms are never recognised, but when the symptoms are present, they may be experienced differently by the individual.

Some symptoms of coronary artery disease may include:

- Tightness, heaviness, pressure and/or pain in the chest—behind the breastbone.
- Pains; radiating in the arms, shoulders, jaw, neck, and/or back.
- Shortness of breath.
- Weakness and fatigue.

DIAGNOSIS OF CORONARY ARTERY DISEASE

In addition to a complete medical history and physical examination, diagnostic procedures for coronary artery disease may include one or a combination of the followings:

- Electrocardiogram (ECG or EKG).

- Stress test or exercise ECG.

- Cardiac catheterization (x-rays are taken after a contrast agent is injected into an artery—to locate the narrowing, occlusions, and other abnormalities of specific arteries.

- Nuclear scanning (radioactive material is injected into a vein and then is observed using a camera as it is taken up by the heart muscle, indicating the healthy and damaged areas of the heart.

Specific treatment for coronary artery disease will be determined by the physician based on medical history and overall health, age and progression of the disease. Treatment may also include modification of risk factors such as; smoking, elevated cholesterol levels, elevated blood pressure, poor dietary habits, being overweight, and lack of exercise. Medications and other medical procedures may also be prescribed to treat the disease.

Medications may reportedly include—anti-platelet medications, anti-coagulants, anti-hyperlipidemics and anti-hypertensive drugs; while procedures may include coronary angioplasty or balloon angioplasty.

Heart Attack
(Myocardial Infarction or MI)

A heart attack occurs when one or more areas of the heart muscle experience a serious or prolonged lack of oxygen caused by blocked (occlusion) or restricted (stenosis) blood flow to the heart muscle. The blockage or restriction is often a result of atherosclerosis and a blood clot. The diseased area could rupture and develop a blood clot, comprising blood clotting protein, platelets and red blood cells. The blood clot that forms within the plaque-obstructed area is said to cause the heart attack.

If the blood and oxygen supply is cut off for a prolonged period, muscle cells of the heart may suffer damage and die, resulting in the dysfunction of the affected area.

Warning signs of a heart attack

Symptoms of a heart attack will depend on severity and muscle area affected. Although chest pain is the key warning sign of a heart attack, it may be confused with indigestion or any other disorders. However, each individual may experience symptoms differently. Symptoms may include:

- Indigestion (dyspepsia)—this may manifest as painful or burning feeling in the upper stomach that may include abdominal bloating; belching; vomiting; severe pain in the upper right abdomen; discomfort unrelated to eating and indigestion accompanied by shortness of breath, sweating, or pain radiating to the jaw, neck or arm. The symptoms of indigestion may resemble other medical conditions; therefore, consult with your physician for proper diagnosis.

- Severe pain, squeezing and/or discomfort in the centre of the chest that lasts for more than a few minutes or that spreads to the shoulders, neck, arms or jaw.

- Chest pain that increases in intensity or that is not relieved by rest.

- Chest pain that occurs additionally with; sweating, shortness of breath, nausea or vomiting, dizziness or fainting, and rapid or irregular pulse.

- Unexplained weakness or fatigue.

If any of the associative symptoms is experienced, immediate medical assistance should be sort.

It is also advisable to avoid getting anxious and to rest while awaiting help; and equally important not to drive as the condition might worsen enroute.

The aim of the treatment for a heart attack is initially to relieve the pain, preserve the heart muscle function and ultimately prevent death.

Risk factors for heart attack

A heart attack can happen to anyone and it is only when care is taken to learn more about the applicable risk factors that steps can be taken to reduce or eliminate them. Some of the risk factors might include:

- Inherited or acquired hypertension (high blood pressure).
- Inherited or acquired low levels of HDL, or high levels of LDL, blood cholesterol or high levels of triglycerides.
- Family history of heart disease.
- Smoking.
- Excessive alcohol consumption.
- Diabetes.
- Stress.
- Overweight.
- Lack of exercise.
- Unhealthy eating habits.

Managing ones risk for a heart attack can begin with:

- Examination of applicable risk factors and then taking steps to reduce or eliminate them.
- Becoming aware of conditions like hypertension and abnormal lipid levels.
- Modifying risk factors that are acquired, not inherited, through lifestyle changes.
- Consultation with ones physician to determine how inherited or genetic risk factors, that cannot be changed, may be managed medically and through lifestyle changes.

It is reported that majority of fatal heart attacks occur in the morning on waking and getting out of bed. The burst of adrenaline that accompanies getting out of bed in the morning might just be the last straw if one is at risk and it could be fatal. Adrenaline is the hormone produced by the medulla of the adrenal glands which, amongst other things, is said to be a potent vasopressor. It acts on the cardiovascular system and stimulates the myocardium (heart muscle) to increase cardiac output.

Heart Failure

Heart failure, also known as cardiac decompensation or congestive heart failure, is a condition in which the heart cannot pump enough oxygenated blood to meet the needs of the body's other organs. Normally, the heart has sufficient reserve strength to compensate for handicaps in most disorders; however, as the disorder increases in severity, the heart muscle becomes more fatigued and increasingly incapable of meeting its pumping obligations. The heart keeps pumping, but not as efficiently as a healthy heart and the loss of pumping action is an indication of an underlying heart problem.

Heart failure may affect the left (left ventricular failure), right (right ventricular failure), or both sides of the heart (bi-ventricular failure). If the left half is affected, fluid will build up in the lungs due to congestion of the veins of the lungs. And if the right half of the heart fails, general body vein pressure will increase, resulting in fluid accumulation in the body—especially leg tissues and abdominal organs. The liver and kidneys might also be affected. Often, left heart failure is said to lead to right failure and causing bi-ventricular failure.

Heart failure is also said to interfere with the kidney's normal function of eliminating excess salt and waste from the body. And in congestive heart failure, the body retains more fluid; resulting in the swelling of the ankles and legs, while fluid also collects in the lungs resulting in shortness of breath.

SYMPTOMS

Symptoms of heart failure and severity of the condition depends on how much of the heart's pumping capacity has been lost. Symptoms may include:

- Shortness of breath during rest, exercise or lying flat with mobility difficulty.
- Breathing problems occurring upon excersion and increasing to breathlessness at rest.
- Waking up breathless at night.

- Fatigue and weakness.
- Loss of appetite and nausea.
- Persistent cough—often with frothy or blood-tinged sputum.
- Weight gain.
- Visible swelling of the legs (oedema) and ankles.
- Reduced urination.
- Possible accumulation of fluid in the abdominal cavity and organs.
- Possible liver enlargement.
- Dry, scaly skin on lower legs and venous leg ulcers resulting from eczema-type rash.
- Possible scrotum enlargement in men.

The symptoms of heart failure may resemble many other conditions or medical problems, so always consult your doctor for a diagnosis and treatment.

RISK FACTORS AND CAUSES

Heart failure can be progressive with the potential for gradual deterioration but treatment can slow the progression of the disease. It can also be a sudden, acute, or chronic long-standing condition. Risk factors and primary causes may include:

- Smoking.
- Overweight.
- Lack of exercise.
- Unhealthy eating habit.
- High blood pressure (hypertension).
- High blood cholesterol.
- Heart valve diseases-caused by previous rheumatic fever or other infections.
- Chronic heart muscle disease.
- Congenital heart disease or defects (present at birth).

- Coronary artery disease or atherosclerosis—narrowed arteries that supply blood to the heart.
- Previous heart attack(s)—scar tissue from previous attacks may interfere with the heart muscle's ability to function normally.
- Endocrine system disorders.
- Cardiac arrhythmias (irregular heart beats).
- Chronic lung disease and pulmonary embolism.
- Drug-induced heart failure.
- Anaemia and haemorrhage.
- Excessive salt intake.
- Diabetes.

Treatment for heart failure

The cause of the heart failure and extent of damage will dictate the treatment regime and specific treatment will be determined by the physician based on—medical history; extent of the disease; age; overall health; and tolerance for a specific medication, procedures, or therapies.

The goal of the treatment is to improve the patient's quality of life through appropriate lifestyle changes and implementing drug therapy. Although there is no cure for heart failure due to a damaged heart muscle, many forms of treatment have proven to be successful.

Lifestyle changes to reduce heart failure risk factors may include:

- Avoiding smoking.
- Weight reduction, if overweight.
- Exercise regularly.
- Eating a healthy, low-fat diet.
- Immediate treatment of any disease that increases the risk of heart failure.

In addition to a complete medical history and physical examination; diagnostic procedures for heart failure may include any, or a combination of, the following procedures:

- Chest x-ray.
- Electrocardiogram (ECG or EKG).
- Echocardiogram—a non-evasive test, using sound waves to produce a study of the motion of the heart's chambers and valves.
- BNP testing—B-type natriuretic peptide (BNP) is said to be a hormone that is released from the ventricles in response to increased wall tension (stress) that occurs with heart failure. BNP levels rise as wall stress increases and is therefore useful in the rapid evaluation of heart failure. The higher the BNP levels, the worse the heart failure condition.

Angina

Angina is a cardiovascular disease of pain in the chest that is often brought on by excersion. It feels like an oppressive, heavy, crushing pain or constricting feeling in the centre of the chest behind the breastbone (sternum) or on the left side of the frontal chest. The pain can radiate out to either one or both arms, more likely the left. It may also be experienced in the jaws, throat, stomach, or between the shoulder blades. But once the trigger factor stops, the pain generally reduces quickly, usually within two to ten minutes.

Trigger factors can include; physical excersion, extreme cold or windy weather condition, a heavy meal, and psychological stress.

Symptoms of angina may also include—increased shortness of breath during exercise (even briefly, such as walking); sense of heaviness or numbness in the arm, shoulder, elbow or hand (usually the left side); a constricting sensation in the throat; weakness and/or fatigue.

CAUSES AND RISK FACTORS

The primary cause of angina is coronary atherosclerosis. Coronary arteries supply the cardiac muscle with blood carrying oxygen and nutrients. Narrow coronary arteries reduce blood flow to the heart muscle, and the effect is usually more noticeable when the heart needs more blood supply, such as during physical activity. With increasing workload, the heart muscles will receive too little oxygen, resulting in stress which then causes pain in the heart. In severe cases the pain can also be felt when the body is at rest or in the morning, on waking and getting out of bed.

Other secondary causes might include:

- Anaemia.
- Heart valve diseases.

- Thickening of the heart muscle (hypertrophy); this can be caused by sustained high blood pressure.

- Sustained fast heart beat.

Risk factors for angina may include:

- Family history of atherosclerosis.

- High blood LDL cholesterol.

- High blood pressure.

- Smoking.

- Diabetes.

- Overweight.

- Stress.

- Lack of regular exercise.

- Being male.

Actions that can be taken to eliminate the risk factors of angina may include:

- Eating a varied and healthy diet, including—leafy vegetables; unprocessed cereals; low-fat, high-fibre foods; and avoiding saturated fats and salts.

- Stop smoking.

- Lose weight—if overweight.

- Exercise more.

- Attend to medical conditions such as atherosclerosis, high blood pressure and diabetes.

- Reduce stress by avoiding stressful situations or adopt different relaxation techniques.

If any associative symptoms of angina are experienced, immediately consult your doctor and follow his advice.

Diagnosing angina

In addition to the patient's medical history and examination, the physician can often diagnose angina by noting the symptoms and frequency of occurrence. Certain diagnostic procedures may also be used to determine the severity of the underlying coronary heart disease, and may include:

- Electrocardiogram (ECG or EKG).

- Stress test (exercise ECG).

- Cardiac catheterization—with this procedure, x-rays are taken after a contrast agent is injected into an artery to locate the narrowing, occlusions, and other possible abnormalities of the specific artery.

TREATMENT OF ANGINA

Treatment of angina will be determined by the physician based on the patient's medical history; overall health; age; extent of the disease; and tolerance for specific medications, procedures, or therapies.

Also, the underlying coronary artery disease that causes the angina should be treated by controlling existing risk factors.

Medications may be prescribed for patients with angina. The reportedly most common medication is nitroglycerin, which helps to relieve pain by widening the blood vessels. This allows more blood flow to the heart muscle and decreases the workload of the heart.

Advice on control or avoidance of some of the trigger factors may also be given, including:

- Rest or engage in quiet activity after a large or heavy meal—the body diverts extra blood flow to the digestive system to aid digestion, so the heart receives less oxygen and is vulnerable to an attack.

- Avoid or seek protection from cold or windy condition—cold air stimulates muscular reflexes that can cause an attack of angina.

- Avoid stressful situations.

- Avoid sudden strenuous moves or lifting heavy objects.

Stroke

Stroke or Cerebrovascular Accidents (CVA); is a cardiovascular disease that occurs when the blood supply to the brain is disturbed in some ways, resulting in brain cells being starved of oxygen and nutrients causing some cells to die or be damaged. Stroke can be caused either by an obstruction of blood flow to the brain or by a blood vessel rupturing and preventing blood flow to the brain.

Types of Stroke

Strokes can be classified into two main categories:

- Ischemic strokes; and
- Hemorrhagic strokes.

Ischemic strokes

This occurs as a result of obstruction within a blood vessel supplying blood to the brain and the underlying condition for this type of stoke is atherosclerosis (a build-up of fat and lipids inside the walls of the blood vessels). Ischemic strokes are further divided into the followings:

- Transient ischemic attacks (TIAs)—these are minor or warning strokes. TIAs may last from a few minutes to a few days and are often a warning sign that a stroke may occur. Although usually mild and transient, the symptoms are similar to those caused by a typical stroke; the obstructive blood clot occurs for a short time and tends to resolve itself through normal body mechanisms.

- Thrombotic strokes are strokes caused by a thrombus (blood clot) that develops in the arteries supplying blood to the brain. This type of stroke is said to be seen usually in older persons, especially those with high cholesterol levels and atherosclerosis.

- Embolic strokes are strokes that are usually caused by an embolus. This is a blood clot that forms at another location in the circulatory system and travels through the blood stream to the brain. Embolic strokes is said to often result from heart disease or heart surgery and can occur rapidly, without any warning signs.

Hemorrhagic strokes

This type of stroke is said to occur when a blood vessel that supplies the brain ruptures and bleeds. When an artery bleeds into the brain, the cells and tissues do not receive oxygen and nutrients; additionally, pressure builds up in the surrounding tissues, causing swelling and irritation.

The two types of hemorrhagic strokes are; intracerebral hemorrhage and subarachnoid hemorrhage.

- Intracerebral hemorrhage is bleeding from the blood vessels within the brain. The bleeding occurs suddenly and rapidly; usually with no warning signs and can be severe enough to cause coma or death. It is said to be caused usually by hypertension (high blood pressure).

- Subarachnoid hemorrhage is bleeding in the subarachnoid space. This results when bleeding occurs between the brain and the meninges (the membrane that covers the brain) in the subarachnoid space. Subarachnoid hemorrhage is said to be often due to an aneurysm or an arteriovenous malformation (AVM). An aneurysm is a weakened, ballooned area of an artery wall and has a risk of rupturing. It may be congenital (present at birth), or may develop later in life due to such factors as hypertension or atherosclerosis. An AVM is a congenital disorder that is said to consist of a disorderly tangled web of arteries and veins. Any of these vessels can rupture and bleed into the brain. The cause of AVM is still unknown.

Recurrent strokes is said to occur in about twenty-five percent of stroke victims within five years after the first attack. The risk is reportedly greatest right after a stroke and decreases over time, with the likelihood of severe disability and death increasing with each recurrent stroke. Furthermore, it is also reported that about three percent of stroke victims have a second attack within thirty days of the first stroke, and one-third have a second stroke within two years. This is quite alarming and underscores the need for continuous monitoring, treatment and reduction of risk factors, especially when someone has shown symptoms of a stroke or had an attack.

Effects of Stroke

The brain is a very complex organ that controls several body functions, and if a stroke occurs and blood flow is interrupted to a region that controls a particular body function, that part will not work as it should.

The effects of a stroke depend on several factors including the location of the obstruction and how much brain tissue is affected. However, since one side of the brain controls the opposite side of the body, a stroke affecting one side will result in neurological complications on the body side it controls. If the stroke occurs in the right side of the brain, then the left side of the body (and the right face side) will be affected; producing any or all of the followings:—paralysis on the left side of the body; vision problems; quick inquisitive behavioural style; and memory loss.

If the stroke occurs in the left side of the brain, the right side of the body (and the left face side) will be affected; producing some or all of the followings:—paralysis on the right side of the body; speech/language problems; slow, cautious behavioural style; and memory loss.

If the stroke occurs towards the back of the brain, it's likely that some disability involving vision will result.

Reducing Risk Factors

Both coronary heart disease and stroke are reported to share common risk factors. Most of them can be modified, treated or controlled while some cannot. Some of the risk factors include:—

- High blood pressure (hypertension).

- Smoking.

- Cholesterol disorders—(high blood LDL, low blood HDL).

- Diabetes.

- Excessive alcohol intake.

- Physical inactivity.

- History of atherosclerosis.

- Being overweight or obese.

- Irregular heart beat (artrial fibrillation—fairly common in old age).

Controlling the risk factors with lifestyle changes; and with prescribed, supervised medication aimed at controlling some underlying factors, the onset of stroke can be retarded.

Treatments for stroke

Stroke is said to be a medical emergency. Knowing the warning signs and calling for medical assistance immediately can save lives, because time lost is brain lost. Since their mechanisms are different, the treatments for the types of strokes are different. When someone has shown symptoms of a stroke or TIA, the doctor will gather information, make a diagnosis and chart a course of treatment.

After the initial emergency treatment, health professionals will focus on preventing complications and future strokes. The patient will also be involved in a stroke rehabilitation programme as soon as possible.

Symptoms of Stroke

Symptoms of a stroke is said to begin suddenly and may include the followings:

- Sudden weakness, numbness or paralysis of the face, arm, or leg; especially on one side of the body.
- Sudden vision problems in one or both eyes, such as double or loss of vision.
- Confusion, with speech or comprehension problems.
- Trouble walking, dizziness, loss of balance or coordination.
- Sudden, severe headache with no known cause.

A prompt action is crucial with the indication or recognition of any stoke associative symptom. Seek immediate medical assistance since every seconds count.

Part Four:

Some Diagnostic Tests and Checks

Cholesterol

Cholesterol is a fatty substance contained in certain foods we eat and also produced in the liver and therefore found in the chemical analysis of the blood. Cholesterol and another lipid, triglyceride, are important building blocks in the cell structure and are also used in making hormones and producing energy. It is also reported to be one of the disease fighting substances in the body; so when the arterial walls are damaged, the body's response is to try and repair the damage by slapping on patches of cholesterol.

Cholesterol is the actual material deposition in the blood vessels during hardening of the arteries (arteriosclerosis). Blood level cholesterol is not solely dependent upon what we eat but also on how the body makes cholesterol in the liver. It is thought that high cholesterol level tend towards premature arteriosclerosis. Cholesterol levels vary markedly in different people. Animal fat is reported to increase cholesterol level while vegetable fat do not seem to cause much harm or elevate blood cholesterol, but unfortunately, decline in the blood cholesterol level by a low-fat, low-cholesterol diet alone does not always occur as the body produces its own cholesterol.

There are two identified sorts of cholesterol:—High density lipoprotein (HDL)—good sort, and Low density lipoprotein (LDL)—bad sort.

HDL—is reported to actually protect against arteriosclerosis by reducing tissue cholesterol and taking it back to the lever, where it is removed and passed from the body. It also removes excess cholesterol from plaques and thus slows their growth. Its level can be raised by exercising.

LDL—is the major cholesterol carrier in the blood and is reported to contribute to diseases of the arteries (cardiovascular diseases). If there is too much of this cholesterol circulating in the blood, it can slowly build up on the artery walls forming plaque. LDL level can be lowered by eating a low-fat diet and medication.

It is the proportion of HDL cholesterol to LDL cholesterol that influences the degree to which arteriosclerosis is likely to cause problems (risk factor).

Triglyceride

Triglyceride:—this ordinarily means fat within the body. The blood contains a certain amount of fat in circulation and most people with elevated triglyceride level in the blood are generally over weight. It is also a contributory lipid that forms part of the building block in the body cell structure and used in making hormones and producing energy. Normal level is 30-175mg per 100cc. The best recommended treatment for elevated level is weight loss.

Homocysteine

Homocysteine:—a reported newly identified cause of clogged arteries is a substance called Homocysteine. It is believed to lead the attack on the artery walls by converting cholesterol into oxidised LDL cholesterol, a far more dangerous form, which attacks artery walls. As the arteries become damaged, other cells stick to it until they become clogged, thickened and less flexible. Homocysteine is also reported to make the blood clot more easily and more likely to form a blockage in the arteries or the organ it supplies.

Lipid (lipoprotein) Profile Tests

This is a group of tests that are often requested together to determine the risk of coronary heart disease. They have been shown to be good indicators as to if someone is likely to have a heart attack or stroke caused by blood vessel blockage and hardening of the arteries.

The lipoprotein profile tests include—Total cholesterol, HDL cholesterol (good), LDL cholesterol (bad), and Triglyceride tests. After a 12—hour fast during which only water is consumed; a blood sample is taken to measure the cholesterol values in the blood. The report may include additional calculated values such as HDL/total cholesterol ratio, HDL/LDL ratio or a risk score based on lipid profile results, age, sex, and other risk factors.

The lipid profile is used in deciding how a person at risk should be treated. The results are considered along with other known risk factors of heart disease to develop a plan of treatment and follow up. Further evidence of cardiovascular disease may also be carried out by checking the pulse, blood pressure, listening to the heart beat/large arteries, checking kidney function via blood test, and arranging ECG (electrocardiogram).

TOTAL CHOLESTEROL COUNT

Total cholesterol count:—High blood cholesterol has been associated with hardening of the arteries, heart disease and risk of heart attack. Cholesterol level testing is used to estimate risk of developing heart disease. It is also considered a routine part of preventive healthcare particularly in persons already with heart disease; family history of high blood cholesterol; over 35 years and with diabetes and high blood pressure; smoker; and those already taking cholesterol lowering drugs.

The target value of total cholesterol should be less than 200 mg/dL, which is measured in milligrams (mg) of cholesterol per decilitre (dL) of blood. 200-239 mg/dL is said to be borderline high, and 240 mg/dL or more is high.

The measured value will be considered with other risk factors for heart disease and this assessment will be used by the doctor to decide on requirement for further treatment in form of dietary changes or drugs to lower the value. However, it is now recognised that the significance of any particular cholesterol level cannot be assessed without taking into account the ratio between HDL and LDL cholesterol or the presence of other cardiovascular risks, such as smoking, diabetes and high blood pressure.

High cholesterol reading can also be due to inherited or familial high cholesterol. Levels can also be influenced by regional origin; with higher levels reported in Northern European countries than in the South and much higher in Asia. Off course, it is known that the relationship to local food is significant and there is also the genes factor. High cholesterol is also seen in connection with other diseases, such as reduced metabolism (Thyroid hormone problems), kidney diseases, diabetes, and alcohol abuse.

LDL (BAD) CHOLESTEROL COUNT

LDL (bad) cholesterol count:—used to determine and predict the risk of developing heart disease. Treatment decisions are often based on LDL values. Elevated levels also known as hyper cholesterolaemia indicates a high risk. Dietary or drug treatment aimed at lowering LDL cholesterol to a target value of less than 100 mg/dL is then initiated.

HDL (GOOD) CHOLESTEROL COUNT

HDL (good) cholesterol count:—used to determine the risk of developing heart disease and as part of regular health check; particularly if one is with a family history of cholesterol disorder, high blood pressure, heart attack, over weight, diabetes, and a smoker. If high cholesterol is due to high HDL, then a person is probably at low risk and no further testing or treatment for high cholesterol is advised.

High HDL is better than low LDL. There are two ways that HDL values are interpreted; either as a measured value or percentage of total cholesterol. When expressed as a ratio of cholesterol to HDL, it is desirable for the ratio to be less than 5. As a value, a good level of HDL is 60 mg/dL or more and this is associated with a less than average risk of heart disease.

Triglycerides Test (TG; TRIG)

This is used to assess the increased risk of developing heart diseases. Triglyceride level is said to increase significantly when blood sugar is out of control, so for diabetics, it is important to have this test as part of any lipid testing. The test for triglycerides is not often ordered alone since risk of heart disease is based on cholesterol levels not triglycerides, however, lipid profiles including triglycerides are recommended as routine tests to evaluate heart disease risk. Having high lipid levels may increase the risk of developing heart disease and treatment may be given to lower the lipid levels. The type of treatment used may differ depending on whether cholesterol or triglycerides or both are high, and also when triglycerides are very high, it is said that there may be risk of developing pancreatis—inflammation of the pancreas. A triglyceride level of 30-175 mg/cc is considered normal.

Cholesterol and triglycerides are two blood tests that can predict the hardening tendency of the arteries (arteriosclerosis). When either is elevated, arteriosclerosis proceeds more rapidly and when both are low, the case is reversed. Cholesterol and triglycerides are highly influenced by diets. Prevention of arteriosclerosis should start early, though never too late. Lipid levels should be checked; if they are normal then there may be no need for regular checks, but if either or both are high, then treatment will be required and the doctor will want regular checks. However, heart attacks and strokes have been reported in cases even with the reassurance of normal lipid level readings.

Homocysteine test

Homocysteine testing, also known as plasma total homocyst, may be requested as part of cardiac risk assessment and also used to help in investigating people who might be at high risk of heart attack or stroke. It may be useful in patients with family history of heart disease without other known risk factors, and it also shows folate or vitamin b12 deficiency, as blood homocysteine concentration is said to be raised in both conditions.

The role of homocysteine testing is however still controversial because the part it plays in the progression of coronary heart disease has not been fully established. Therefore, there are no established guidelines for homocysteine testing and route screening has not been recommended. However, it has been reported that people with raised homocysteine levels have a much higher risk of heart attack or stroke than those with average levels. Coronary artery blockage, which can lead to heart attack, is also reported to occur with more than double the average frequency in people with homocysteine levels in the highest 25% as compared to those in the lowest 25%. This suggests that measurement of homocysteine maybe an even better indication of who is at risk of having a heart attack or stroke than other tests.

Presently, a direct correlation between homocysteine levels and heart attacks has not been fully established, but there is reported strong evidence of a relationship between homocysteine levels and heart attack or stroke survival rates.

It has recently been reported that folic acid, vitamins b6 and b12 have the greatest effect at breaking down harmful homocysteine from within the body. Foods rich in folic acid includes:—green leafy vegetables, citrus fruits, pulses such as black-eyed beans and chick peas, and whole grain cereals.

It is important to consult with your doctor or healthcare worker before taking any medication or food supplements; interaction of some ingredients can be fatal even if beneficial individually; so be careful. It is also advisable to discuss with your doctor further advancement on Homocysteine study and requirement for its level testing.

Electro Cardiogram (ECG; EKG) Check

An electrocardiogram measures electrical activity within the heart. The electric current for every beat is said to begin in a small area of the heart, and then spreads quickly across the entire organ, causing it to contract, and then relax. The ECG records the path of the current, which may coincide with the heart beat. The electrical stimulus is said to be generated by the sinus node (sinoatrial node or SA node), which is a mass of specialised tissue located in the right atrium (right upper heart chamber). The sinus node generates an electrical stimulus regularly and this travels down through the conduction pathways and causes the heart's lower chambers to contract and pump out blood. The right and left atria (the two upper heart chambers) are stimulated first and contract a short period of time before the right and left ventricles (the two lower heart chambers). As the electrical impulse moves through the heart, the heart muscles contract at an average of about 78 times per minute and each contraction represents one heart beat.

Why ECG is done

ECG is a fast, simple, relatively inexpensive and painless test and is used as part of an initial examination to help the doctor narrow the scope of a diagnostic process or check the heart's function. ECG may be done to obtain a baseline tracing of the heart's function and this baseline tracing may be used later as a comparison with future ECGs, to detect if any changes have occurred. Changes in an ECG from the normal tracing can indicate one or more of several heart-related conditions, however, conditions that are not heart-related may also cause changes in the ECG.

ECG may also be done as part of a work-up schedule prior to a procedure such as surgery to ensure a heart condition does not exist that might cause complications during or after the procedure. And furthermore, to check the effectiveness of certain heart medications and heart-related procedures such as bypass surgery or implanted pacemaker.

How ECG is done

During this check, the patient lies on a sofa table or bed and wire leads (electrodes) will be connected at specific locations on the chest, arms, and legs. The electrodes, which are self-sticking, will adhere to the skin, linking points from the ankles, wrists and chest to a nearby machine that reels out paper tape covered with crawly graph lines, indicating a graphical representation or tracing of the electrical activity within the heart. If part of the heart muscle is damaged or distressed and with many areas sending out signals, the ECG will show abnormal current flow or irregular beats and the injured muscle will produce an abnormal trace. It may also indicate an enlarged heart, a problem with one or more of the heart valves or other types of heart conditions; showing that a patient is at risk. The patient will need to lie very still and not talk during the procedure, as movement or talking may interfere with the tracing.

There are additional ECG procedures which are more involved than the basic ECG. These procedures include the following:

Exercise ECG, or Stress test.

The patient is attached to the ECG machine. However, rather than lying down, the patient exercises by walking on a treadmill or pedalling a stationary bicycle while the ECG is recorded. This test is done to assess changes in the ECG during stress such as exercise.

Continuous or Holster monitoring ECG

This is an ECG recording done over a period of 24hours or more. The electrodes are attached to the patient's chest and connected to a small portable ECG recorder while the patient goes about usual daily activities. There are two types of Holster monitoring: Continuous recording—the ECG is recorded continuously during the entire testing period. Event monitoring—the ECG is recorded only when the patient starts the recording or when symptoms are felt.

Holster monitoring ECG is used to further evaluate specific heart condition or when a resting ECG is not conclusive.

Part Five:

Keeping your heart healthy

Keeping your heart healthy

There are a lot that can be done to keep the heart healthy at whatever age. People with heart diseases are also living longer and more productive lives than ever before as a result of advances in medicine and technology. But prevention is still the best weapon in the fight against heart diseases. Whether one is healthy, at high risk for heart disease, or has survived a heart attack—the guidelines for protecting the heart is still the same.

Get involved in physical activity and exercise

Exercise is said to be any type of physical exertion we perform in order to improve our health, shape or bodies and boost performance. Exercise also improves heart function, lowers blood pressure and cholesterol, and boost energy. The heart is a muscle tissue and needs exercise to keep fit so it can pump blood efficiently with each beat. However, it believed that many people live sedentary lives and do not participate in any leisure-time physical activity. You do not need any special skills or training to be physically active. Walking is said to be a great way to be active.

Physical activity should be initiated slowly, and the intensity should be gradually increased to the recommended amount (at least 30 minutes most days). Activities can be split into several short periods (10 minutes, 3 times a day) instead of one longer period (30 minutes once a day). The best exercise is the one you enjoy and can fit into your daily life. Many forms of physical activity can be social—allowing you to spend time with family or friends or to develop new relationships. You can also involve family and friends and support those trying to be physically active.

It may take more time to incorporate more activities into your daily life, but you can start with; parking farther away from the shops or the office to create a longer walk, taking the stairs, walking around the mall when shopping, and walking around the neighbourhood.

Discuss with your doctor what form of exercise is best for you. People with severe heart disease are advised against strenuous exercise.

Cardiovascular exercise is an activity that raises your heart rate to a level where you are working out, but can still talk. Vigorous exercise like running or doing aerobics brings more health benefits than lighter intensity activities; getting your heart rate up and giving you a good workout. During moderate exercise you should be breathing more heavily than normal and feel slightly warmer or sweating. Cardiovascular exercise is said to be important for a healthy heart and weight loss and have the following benefits:

- It makes your heart strong so that it doesn't have to work as hard to pump blood.

- It increases your lung capacity.

- It helps reduce the risk of heart attack, high cholesterol, high blood pressure and diabetes.

- It makes you feel good and helps you sleep better.

- It helps to reduce stress (anxiety and depression).

- It helps to slow bone loss associated with advancing age.

Cardiovascular workouts can be done at home or outdoors, with or without equipment. It involves continuous movements like stair climbing, fast walking, cycling, running, rowing, swimming, and aerobics.

The heart is a muscle tissue and like all body muscles, it requires exercise to keep fit and remain efficient. Cardiovascular exercise works out the heart, thereby helping it meet its obligation.

Some physical activity and exercise start up ideas can be to:

- Start with five minutes exercise at least three times a day, starting slowly at a level that suits you.

- Gradually build up time and frequency until 30 minutes feels easier.

- Choose a variety of activities and ones you enjoy.

- Try to do something everyday.

Note:—Please stop exercising if any pain or discomfort is felt and consult your doctor.

Children and exercise

It is important to involve children in physical activities and teach them early that exercise is fun and good for them. Families can walk together, ride bicycles, and chase after balls in the park.

Some parents-children activity ideas can include:

- Ask children what activities they enjoy and encourage them to do it and participate with them.
- Spend time playing active games with them.
- Provide them with sports equipments to use and participate with them.
- Encourage them to spend time outdoors (mindful of safety oversight).
- Encourage them to walk to school with friends (reasonable distance and where safety is not an issue).
- Try some regular family activities.
- Praise and encourage them as they participate and progress.
- Be a good role model and show them you also enjoy and value physical activities.

Encourage children to be heart healthy conscious.

Overweight and obesity—Maintaining a healthy weight

Weight gain can happen over the years. Generic differences can cause some to gain weight more than others, while certain medical conditions and drugs are also said to be contributory to weight gain. It is advisable to aim for, and cultivate a healthy weight for life. Body Mass Index (BMI) is used to classify overweight and obesity.

BMI (Body Mass Index)

BMI (Body Mass Index)—It was reported that an expert panel, convened by the National Institute of Health (USA) in 1998, recommended its use. BMI is said to correlate with the risk of disease and death (heart disease increases with increasing BMI in all population group); BMI is simple, rapid, and inexpensive to calculate; BMI correlates well with total body fat for the majority of people.

CALCULATING BMI

Calculating BMI—This is a measure of weight in relation to height.

- BMI = weight (kg)/height (metres, squared) or
- BMI = (weight (pounds)/height (inches, squared)) x 703.

Tables to determine BMI are also commonly available.

Generally, a healthy weight is said to fall within the range of 18.5-24.9 index, overweight 25-29.9, and obesity 30 and above.

LIMITATIONS

Limitations—BMI is said to have some limitations in that it can overestimate body fat in persons who are very muscular, and underestimate body fat in persons who have lost muscle mass, such as the elderly.

Solely having a BMI in the overweight or obese range does not necessarily mean that a person is unhealthy. Other risk factors are important to consider when assessing overall health and an actual diagnosis of overweight or obesity should be made by a health professional.

How to loose weight

How to loose weight: Being physically active can help you attain or maintain a healthy weight, especially when it is combined with calorie reduction. Advisably;

- It is important to set a goal (expectation) or desirable result, and focus on achieving it.

- Create healthier eating habits. Follow the recommended Dietary Guidelines. It is reported that reducing your calorie intake by about 150 calories a day, along with participating in moderate activity, could double your weight loss and is equivalent to approximately ten pounds in six months and twenty pounds in one year.

- Serve or eat smaller portions of meal, instead of complete starvation followed by feeding frenzy.

- Increase your everyday activity to balance the calories you consume. You must use more energy than you consume in order to loose weight.

The health consequences of being overweight or obese can be said to include the followings:

- The incidence of heart disease is said to be higher in persons who are overweight or obese (BMI greater than 25). It is also associated with certain types of cancer, type 2 diabetes, stroke, arthritis, breathing problems, and some psychological disorders such as depression.

- High blood pressure is more common in adults who are overweight or obese than those with healthy weight.

- Obesity is associated with elevated triglycerides (body fat) and decreased HDL (good) cholesterol.

- The higher a person's BMI is above 25, the greater is said to be their weight-related health risks.

The benefits of losing weight

The benefits of losing weight may include:

- Lowering the LDL (bad) cholesterol and triglycerides levels.
- Increasing the HDL (good) cholesterol level.
- Reducing blood pressure level.
- Making mobility easier and improving breathing. The extra weight itself may lead to wear and tear on joints, causing symptoms such as pain and breathlessness.
- Lower risk of type 2 diabetes.
- Help sleeping better at night.
- Reducing the strain on the heart.

Maintain a nutritious and well-balanced diet

A healthy diet is said to be one that is low in fat, cholesterol, salt, and sugar; and high in fruits, vegetables, grains, and fibre. It is advisable to select sensible portions and follow recommended dietary guidelines. It is also said that heart-healthy diet should be the routine, so that when you have a high-fat food every now and then, you are still on track.

Like exercise, good eating habits should start early and it is said that teaching children to eat well is one of the most loving things that can be done for them.

Eating oily fish is said to help reduce risk of heart disease. The omega 3 fatty acid it contains reportedly may help keep the heart-beat regular, reduce triglyceride levels, and prevent blood clots forming in the arteries. Salt reduction is said to help keep blood pressure down. Excessive alcohol consumption is said to cause damage to the heart muscle, increase blood pressure, and lead to weight gain.

Fruits are reported to have many nutritional benefits. Their high levels of anti-oxidants, vitamin C, vitamin E, and carotenoids make them a natural and all round healthy preventatives against heart disease and some forms of cancer. However, for some reasons eating fruits feel like an effort. Make it easy and fun—buy an attractive colourful mix of fruits and keep some in a bowl on your desk, dinning table, and kitchen. When someone feels like a snack, take a bite of a sweet and crisp fruit.

Garlic is reported to be a vasodilator, (amongst other things), which causes blood vessels to expand and blood pressure to drop. It is said to improve blood flow in the coronary arteries and throughout the body and also appear to improve the flexibility of the arteries. It is thought that one to two cloves of raw or lightly-cooked garlic a day are probably enough to obtain most of its benefits. But if one cannot stand the powerful aroma and taste, then one can take the enteric-coated garlic supplements. Always consult your doctor before taking any food supplements.

Healthy and nourishing diet is said to help keep a healthy heart by:

- Maintaining a healthy weight, thereby reducing the strain on the heart.
- Lowering blood LDL cholesterol level and increasing the HDL level.
- Keeping blood pressure down.
- Prevent atherosclerosis within the arteries.
- Prevent abnormal clotting of the blood.

Control your blood cholesterol

As with blood pressure, eating a low-fat, low-cholesterol diet and engaging in moderate physical activity can lower cholesterol levels. The body turns saturated fat into cholesterol and the higher the level, the more likely it is that it will build up and stick to the artery walls. Exercising is said to help convert cholesterol into HDL (good) cholesterol. The only way to find out one's cholesterol level is to visit the doctor and have a blood cholesterol test. A lipid profile test will reveal total cholesterol level. Total cholesterol of less than 200 mg/dL is said to be desirable, 200-239 mg/dL is borderline high, and 240 mg/dL or more is high.

Low-density lipoprotein (LDL), also known as "bad cholesterol", should be less than 100 mg/dL.

High-density lipoprotein (HDL), also known as "good cholesterol", protects the heart from bad cholesterol build up, so the higher, the better. HDL of 60 mg/dL or more helps lower heart disease risk.

If lifestyle changes alone do not affect cholesterol levels, then medications may be needed.

Prevent and manage diabetes

Diabetes and heart disease co-exist and heart disease is said to be the leading cause of death in those with diabetes. Diabetes is a disease in which the body does not properly produce or use insulin. Insulin is a hormone needed by the body to convert sugar, starches, and other nutrients into energy. Pre-diabetes is said to exist when blood glucose levels are higher than normal, but not high enough to be diagnosed as diabetes. People can have diabetes without knowing they have it. Genetics and lifestyle factors such as physical inactivity and obesity can lead to diabetes.

Symptoms of diabetes may include the followings:

- Frequent urination.
- Excessive thirst.
- Unusual weight loss.
- Increased fatigue.
- Unusually extreme hunger.
- Irritability.
- Blurry vision.

However, these symptoms are not exclusively for diabetes, and it is advisable to consult a doctor with any of the symptoms for diagnosis.

Control your blood pressure

It is reported that poor eating habits and physical inactivity both contribute to high blood pressure and also that table salt increases average levels of blood pressure. However, this effect is greater in some people than in others. It is important to keep on top of one's blood pressure levels through regular visits to the doctor. If lifestyle changes alone do not bring down the blood pressure to within desirable range, then medications may also be needed.

Quit smoking

Avoiding smoking is said to dramatically lower heart attack risk. And if you do not smoke, do not start. Along with raising the risk of lung cancer and other diseases, the mixture of tar, nicotine, and carbon monoxide in tobacco smoke is said to increase the risk of hardened arteries, which will restrict blood flow to the heart. Therefore, smokers are believed to have more than twice the risk of having a heart attack as non-smokers.

Part Six:

Stress

Stress

Stress is sometimes used to describe the way we feel when under intense pressure or the feeling that is created when we react to particular events or the very fast pace of life that many people live. We all find different things stressful and can experience different signs and symptoms as a result.

The events that provoke stress are called stressors, and they cover a whole range of situations—from outright physical danger to making a speech. The human body responds to stressors by activating the nervous system and specific hormones. The hypothalamus (part of the gray matter in the floor and walls of the third ventricle of the brain) is said to signal the adrenal glands (two small ductless glands over the kidneys) to produce more of the hormones adrenaline and cortisol and release them into the bloodstream. These hormones speed up the heart rate, breathing rate, blood pressure, and metabolism. Blood vessels open wider to let more blood flow to large muscle groups, putting our muscles on alert. Pupils dilate to improve vision. The liver releases some of its stored glucose to increase the body's energy. And sweat is produced to cool the body. All of these physical changes prepare the body to react quickly and effectively to handle the pressure of the moment. This is the fight or flight mode and is known as the stress response.

When working properly, the body's stress response enhances a person's ability to perform well under pressure. But the stress response can also cause problems when it overreacts or fails to turn off and reset itself properly. Long-term stressful situations can produce a lasting, low level stress that's hard on people. The nervous system senses continued pressure and may remain slightly activated and continue to pump out extra stress hormones over an extended period. This can wear out the body's reserve, leave a person feeling depleted or overwhelmed, weaken the body's immune system, and cause other problems.

The link between stress and heart disease is said to be completely unclear, but it is known that stress speeds up the heart rate. Unless there is an underlying condition, stress alone will not cause a heart attack. However, people with heart disease are more likely to have a heart attack during times of stress.

A degree of stress is necessary for us to feel motivated and enthusiastic. Getting it right helps us to lead a healthy, active lifestyle and cope with stress in a positive way. However, coping with stress by employing a temporary fix solution such as too much alcohol, over-eating, or smoking can be unhealthy.

Signs of stress overload

Everyone experiences stress a little differently, and some people under stress overload may experience the followings:

- Anxiety or panic attacks.
- Irritability and moodiness.
- Feeling of being constantly pressured, hurried, and hassled.
- Drinking too much alcohol, smoking, overeating, or doing drugs.
- Sleeping problems.
- Physical symptoms such as stomach problems, headaches, or chest pain.
- Sadness or depression.

Keeping stress under control

What can be done to deal with stress overload or avoid stress in the first place? The most helpful method of dealing with stress is learning how to manage it. Stress-management skills work better when they are used regularly, not just when the pressure is on.

Here are some of the things that can help keep stress under control:

- Learn to relax. Building relaxation into your lifestyle will help cope better with stress and help maintain healthy habits. The body's natural antidote to stress is called the "relaxation response". It is the body's opposite of stress, and it creates a sense of well-being and calm. You can trigger the relaxation mode by using simple breathing exercises when in a stressful situation. Ensure you stay relaxed by building time into your schedule for calming down and for pleasurable activities such as reading a good book; making time for a hobby; spending time with your pet; or taking a relaxing bath.

- Treat your body well. It is believed that getting regular exercise helps people manage stress.

- Get a good night's sleep. Getting enough sleep helps keep your body and mind in top shape and makes you better equipped to deal with any negative stress.

- Be realistic—do not try to be perfect and do not expect others to be perfect.

- Take a stand against over scheduling.

- Solve the little problems—learning to solve everyday little problems can give you a sense of control.

Treating Heart Disease

Once your doctor has concluded that you have coronary artery disease, the treatment plan would typically involve a combination of drugs, lifestyle changes, and procedures that open up the arteries.

Drugs:—clot-dissolving drugs (thrombolytic drugs) are given during heart attack treatment to dissolve the blood clots in the coronary arteries and restore blood flow to the heart. Due to its anti-clotting abilities, aspirin is reported to have been recognised as safe and effective to help lower the risk of having a second heart attack. There are gastro-resistant (enteric coated) versions of aspirin that are non-irritant to the stomach.

Other drugs that are used to treat people with heart disease include drugs that lower blood pressure; drugs that help the heart pump better (angiotensin-converting (ACE) inhibitors); and beta blockers, which slow the heart down. Nitrates and calcium channel blockers are said to relax the blood vessels and relieve chest pain. Diuretics decrease fluid retention in the body. Blood cholesterol-lowering drugs reduce levels of low-density lipoproteins (LDL), the bad cholesterol in the blood and increase the high-density lipoproteins (HDL), the good cholesterol.

Catheter-based treatments:—Angioplasty is a procedure where by a thin tube (catheter) is put into the artery in the groin and threaded up to the narrowed artery in the heart. The catheter, which has a balloon at the tip, is used to widen the artery.

Coronary bypass surgery:—In case of severe blockages or when a patient is unresponsive to medication or not a candidate for angioplasty, doctors may perform coronary bypass surgery. This involves taking a blood vessel from the leg or chest and grafting it into the blocked artery to bypass the blockage.

Conclusion

Eating a nutritious and well-balanced diet combined with the recommended amount of physical activity (thirty minutes of moderate activity on at least five days a week), is said to help lower the risk of coronary artery disease, cardiovascular disease, and other related diseases. It also gives more energy and stamina, improves the feeling of well-being, as well as helps to better cope with stress.

It is recommended that as an adult, everyone should know their numbers. Get a lipoprotein profile test and find out what their total cholesterol, LDL cholesterol, HDL cholesterol, and triglyceride numbers are. Know your blood pressure. Know your body mass index (BMI) and see how your weight measures up. Discuss your risk for heart disease with your doctor or health care worker and take steps to reduce the controllable risk factors and ensure your numbers are within the desirable range.

Prevention is still the best weapon in the fight against cardiovascular and coronary artery diseases.

About the Author

Gabriel Ademola is a flight engineer, operating as part of a flight deck crew with a UK based cargo airline. He currently resides in Lagos, Nigeria with his wife and children. He has travelled world-wide and interacted with different people. Gabriel has also gone through series of medical checks, as a requirement for flight crew licence renewals. His interaction with different doctors and healthcare personnel and the experiences of some loved ones and friends prompted the interest in and data collection about cardiovascular and coronary artery diseases.

This has been presented in an unbiased view so that everyone can be conscious of the need to start early to protect the heart and blood vessels from the ravages of these diseases. There is the need to modify some of our life styles and choices in order to reduce the risk of developing these diseases and keep our heart and blood vessels healthy.

Resources

www.nhlbi.nih.gov/health/dci/Diseases/sca/SCA
www.health.gov/dietaryguidelines
www.healthsystems.virginia.edu/UVAHealth/adult_cardiacattack.cfm
www.medicalcenter.osu.edu/patientcare/healthcare_services/stroke
www.surgeongeneral.gov/topics/obesity/calltoaction/fact_advice
www.nhlbi.nih.gov/health/hearttruth
www.americanheart.org/simplesolutions
www.kidshealth.org-stress
www.mckinley.uiuc.edu/sickle_cell_disease

978-0-595-51407-6
0-595-51407-3